MCQs in
ANATOMY

Dr. Usha Dhall
Professor & Head, Department of Anatomy,
Postgraduate Institute of Medical Sciences, Rohtak

Dr. J.C. Dhall
Ex Professor & Head, Department of Surgery,
Postgraduate Institute of Medical Sciences, Rohtak

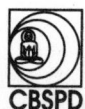

CBSPD

CBS Publishers & Distributors Pvt Ltd

New Delhi • Bengaluru • Chennai • Kochi • Kolkata • Lucknow • Mumbai
Hyderabad • Jharkhand • Nagpur • Patna • Pune • Uttarakhand

MCQs in Anatomy

ISBN: 978-81-239-0906-3

Copyright © Authors and Publisher

Second Edition: 2003
Reprint: 2003, 2004, 2005, 2006, 2007, 2011, 2013, 2015, 2017, 2021, 2023

First Edition: 1992

Published by Satish Kumar Jain and Produced by Varun Jain for

CBS Publishers & Distributors Pvt Ltd
4819/XI Prahlad Street, 24 Ansari Road, Daryaganj, New Delhi 110 002, India.   4819/XI Prahlad Street, 24 Ansari Road, Daryaganj, New Delhi 110 002, India.
Ph: 011-23289259, 23266861   Website: www.cbspd.com
                                    e-mail: delhi@cbspd.com
Corporate Office: 204 FIE, Industrial Area, Patparganj, Delhi 110 092
Ph: 011-4934 4934 Fax: 011-4934 4935   e-mail: publishing@cbspd.com;
                                          publicity@cbspd.com

Branches

- **Bengaluru:** Seema House 2975, 17th Cross, K.R. Road, Banasankari 2nd Stage, Bengaluru 560 070, Karnataka, India
  Ph: +91-80-26771678/79   Fax: +91-80-26771680   e-mail: bangalore@cbspd.com
- **Chennai:** 7, Subbaraya Street, Shenoy Nagar, Chennai 600 030, Tamil Nadu, India
  Ph: +91-44-26680620/26681266   Fax: +91-44-42032115   e-mail: chennai@cbspd.com
- **Kochi:** 42/1325, 1326, Power House Road, Opp KSEB, Power House, Ernakulam 682 018, Kochi, Kerala, India
  Ph: +91-484-4059061-65, 67   Fax: +91-484-4059065   e-mail: kochi@cbspd.com
- **Kolkata:** 147, Hind Ceramics Compound, 1st Floor, Nilgunj Road, Belghoria, Kolkata-700056, West Bengal, India
  Ph: +033-25633055, 033-25633056   e-mail: kolkata@cbspd.com
- **Lucknow:** Basement, Khushnuma Complex, 7 Meerabai Marg (Behind Jawahar Bhawan), Lucknow-226001, UP, India
  Ph: +91-522-4000032   e-mail: tiwari.lucknow@cbspd.com
- **Mumbai:** PWD Shed, Gala no 25/26, Ramchandra Bhatt Marg, Next to JJ Hospital Gate no. 2, Opp. Union Bank of India Noorbaug, Mumbai-400009, Maharashtra, India
  Ph: 022-66661880/89   e-mail: mumbai@cbspd.com

Representatives

• **Hyderabad**	0-9885175004	• **Jharkhand**	0-9811541605	• **Nagpur**	0-94219455˙
• **Patna**	0-9334159340	• **Pune**	0-9923910676	• **Uttarakhand**	0-971646245

Printed at Glorious Printer, Jhilmil Colony, Delhi, India

Preface

In preparing the 2nd edition of this book, I have maintained the overall structure and arrangement of the book. The entire book has undergone a comprehensive revision directed towards greater clarity. Many more questions have been added in each section particularly in relation to Clinical Anatomy keeping in view the latest recommendations of Medical Council of India.

It is hoped that this book will be of use to the students of Anatomy and those preparing for entrance examination for postgraduate degree course in Anatomy, Surgery, Medicine and allied disciplines.

I am grateful to my students, colleagues and friends who inspired me to revise this book. I owe special thanks to Mr. Satish Kalra for help in typing & M/s C.B.S. Publishers and Distributors, Delhi for promptness in bringing up this publication.

Usha Dhall

J.C. Dhall

Contents

PART-I

GROSS ANATOMY

CHAPTER 1

Head and Neck

Directions: Each of the incomplete statements or questions below is followed by four or five suggested completions or answers. Select the one which is BEST in each case.

1. **The point where the frontal bone meets the two parietal bones is called**
   - A. bregma
   - B. lambda
   - C. glabella
   - D. asterion
   - E. pterion

2. **The anterior fontanellae**
   - A. is triangular in shape
   - B. disappears at six months age
   - C. gives an idea of the state of dehydration of the baby
   - D. becomes depressed when the baby cries
   - E. has none of the above features

3. **Mandibular fossa is a part of**
   - A. mandible
   - B. maxilla
   - C. sphenoid bone
   - D. temporal bone
   - E. none of the above bones

4. **Which of the following bones does *not* take part in the formation of floor of temporal fossa?**
   - A. Zygomatic
   - B. Frontal
   - C. Temporal
   - D. Parietal
   - E. Sphenoid

Ans.   1. A   2. C   3. D   4. A

5. **Which of the following bones does *not* contain an air sinus?**
    A. Frontal
    B. Maxilla
    C. Occipital
    D. Temporal
    E. Ethmoid

6. **The mental foramen is usually located**
    A. below the first premolar tooth
    B. between the first and second premolar teeth
    C. below the first molar tooth
    D. between the first and second molar teeth

7. **The dental formula for the milk teeth is**
    A. 2012
    B. 2102
    C. 2132
    D. 2123
    E. none of the above

8. **The first permanent tooth to appear is the**
    A. medial incisor
    B. lateral incisor
    C. first premolar
    D. first molar
    E. canine

9. **The upper molar teeth are supplied by**
    A. lingual nerve
    B. infraorbital nerve
    C. mandibular nerve
    D. middle superior alveolar nerve
    E. posterior superior alveolar nerve

10. **The jugular foramen does *not* transmit the**
    A. inferior petrosal sinus
    B. straight sinus
    C. glossopharyngeal nerve
    D. accessory nerve
    E. vagus nerve

Ans.   5. C   6. B   7. B   8. D   9. E   10. B

11. **The foramen lacerum is present in the**
    A. sphenoid bone
    B. temporal bone
    C. occipital bone
    D. none of the above bones

12. **The anterior ethmoidal canal opens**
    A. at the junction of the floor and medial wall of orbit
    B. at the junction of the roof and medial wall of orbit
    C. in the roof of orbit
    D. in the medial wall of orbit

13. **The inferior nasal concha is a part of**
    A. ethmoid
    B. palatine
    C. maxilla
    D. none of the above bones

14. **The floor of the orbit is formed by the**
    A. maxilla, zygomatic and sphenoid
    B. maxilla, sphenoid and palatine
    C. maxilla, palatine and zygomatic
    D. maxilla and zygomatic only

15. **The two posterior nasal apertures are separated by the**
    A. perpendicular plate of palatine
    B. perpendicular plate of ethmoid
    C. vomer
    D. rostrum of sphenoid

16. **The basiocciput and the basisphenoid fuse with each other**
    A. at birth
    B. around puberty
    C. at 18-25 years
    D. after 40 years
    E. none of the above

17. **Which of the following statements is *not* true for the atlas vertebra?**
    A. It has no body
    B. The posterior arch is longer than the anterior arch

Ans.   11. D   12. B   13. D   14. C   15. C   16. C

C. The spine is bifid
D. The superior articular facets are elongated and concave
E. It articulates with the axis vertebra forming three synovial joints

18. **The thoracic part of vertebral column**
A. shows secondary curvature
B. consists of ten vertebrae
C. permits free rotation
D. contains cauda equina at birth
E. has mamillary processes

19. **Which of the following statements is true for the fifth lumbar vertebra?**
A. The body is the smallest of all the lumbar vertebrae
B. The transverse process encroaches on to the side of the body
C. The distance between the superior articular processes is greater than the distance between inferior articular processes
D. The spine lies at the level of the highest point of iliac crest
E. The vertebral foramen contains conus medullaris

20. **The nucleus pulposus does *not* receive any support from**
A. annulus fibrosus
B. anterior longitudinal ligament
C. posterior longitudinal ligament
D. ligamentum flavum

21. **Which of these foramina does *not* lie in middle cranial fossa?**
A. Foramen rotundum
B. Foramen lacerum
C. Jugular foramen
D. Foramen spinosum

22. **Which of the following dural folds is attached to crista galli?**
A. Tentorium cerebelli
B. Falx cerebri
C. Falx cerebelli
D. Diaphragma sellae

23. **Which of the following statements regarding cavernous sinus is *False*?**
A. Trochlear nerve passes through it

Ans.   17. C   18. C   19. B   20. D   21. C   22. B

   B. Internal carotid artery passes through it
   C. Hypophysis cerebri lies medial to it
   D. Oculomotor runs through its lateral wall

24. **In a case of head injury the person develops "black eye". The haemorrhage has most likely occurred**
   A. just under the skin of the scalp
   B. under the epicranial aponeurosis
   C. under the pericranium
   D. within the cranial cavity

25. **The sternomastoid muscle**
   A. arises from the mastoid process
   B. is inserted into the sternum and the clavicle
   C. is supplied by cranial part of accessory nerve
   D. turns the head to the opposite side
   E. divides the subclavian artery into three parts

26. **The scalenus anterior muscle**
   A. is attached to the posterior tubercles of cervical vertebrae
   B. is related anteriorly to roots of brachial plexus
   C. flexes the vertebral column
   D. separates the subclavian artery from the subclavian vein
   E. is inserted on the second rib

27. **The suboccipital muscles**
   A. include the semispinalis capitis
   B. are all supplied by the dorsal ramus of first cervical nerve
   C. mainly support the vertebral column
   D. are just under cover of the trapezius muscle
   E. lie between atlas and occipital bone

28. **The infrahyoid muscles do *not* include the**
   A. omohyoid
   B. sternohyoid
   C. geniohyoid
   D. sternothyroid
   E. thyrohyoid

29. **The digastric muscle is supplied by**
   A. facial nerve

Ans.   23. A   24. B   25. D   26. D   27. B   28. C

B. mandibular nerve
C. hypoglossal nerve
D. glossopharyngeal and mandibular nerves
E. facial and mandibular nerves

30. **The mylohyoid muscle**
A. forms the floor of oral cavity
B. arises from the mylohyoid groove of mandible
C. is inserted along the whole length of the greater cornu of hyoid bone
D. is related to the submental lymphnodes on its deep surface
E. is supplied by ansa cervicalis

31. **Which of the following muscles does *not* form any boundary of the carotid triangle?**
A. Sternomastoid
B. Omohyoid
C. Sternohyoid
D. Digastric

32. **The main muscular landmark in the neck is the**
A. trapezius
B. sternomastoid
C. digastric
D. omohyoid
E. sternohyoid

33. **The orbicularis oculi is supplied by the**
A. temporal branch of facial nerve
B. supraorbital nerve
C. oculomotor nerve
D. infraorbital nerve
E. zygomatico-facial nerve

34. **The buccinator muscle**
A. takes origin from mandible only
B. forms pharyngeal raphe with superior constrictor of pharynx
C. is supplied by the buccal branch of mandibular nerve
D. is pierced by the parotid duct
E. helps in opening the mouth

Ans.   29. E   30. A   31. C   32. B   33. A   34. D

35. **The nerve supply to stapedius muscle comes from the**
    A. chorda tympani nerve
    B. auricular branch of vagus nerve
    C. direct branch from facial nerve
    D. tympanic branch of glossopharyngeal nerve
    E. carotico-tympanic nerves

36. **Which of the following nerves supplies the platysma?**
    A. Cervical plexus
    B. Facial nerve
    C. Mandibular nerve
    D. Vagus nerve
    E. None of the above

37. **Haemorrhage in the subdural space is most likely due to the rupture of**
    A. diploic veins
    B. superficial temporal artery
    C. cerebral vein
    D. cerebral artery
    E. middle meningeal vein

38. **Which of the following veins is a tributary of the subclavian vein?**
    A. External jugular vein
    B. Vertebral vein
    C. Inferior thyroid vein
    D. Internal thoracic vein

39. **Which of the following is *not* a tributary of the internal jugular vein?**
    A. Inferior petrosal sinus
    B. Inferior thyroid vein
    C. Middle thyroid vein
    D. Lingual vein
    E. Jugular lymph trunk

40. **Which of the following branches of external carotid artery arises just above the level of greater cornu of hyoid bone?**
    A. Lingual artery
    B. Facial artery

Ans.   35. C   36. B   37. C   38. A   39. B

    C. Superior thyroid artery
    D. Ascending pharyngeal artery

41. **Middle meningeal artery is the branch of**
    A. maxillary artery
    B. superficial temporal artery
    C. external carotid artery
    D. internal carotid artery

42. **Inferior thyroid vein terminates into**
    A. internal jugular vein
    B. external jugular vein
    C. anterior jugular vein
    D. brachiocephalic vein

43. **Pulsation of which of the following arteries is *not* normally palpable?**
    A. Common carotid artery
    B. Femoral artery
    C. Axillary artery
    D. Superficial temporal artery

44. **Which of the following arteries is *not* tortuous?**
    A. Ophthalmic
    B. Splenic
    C. Uterine
    D. Vertebral

45. **Which of the following arteries is *not* an end artery?**
    A. Cortical branches of cerebral arteries
    B. Central artery of retina
    C. Segmental branches of renal artery
    D. Segmental branches of splenic artery

46. **Which of the following is *not* a branch of the internal carotid artery?**
    A. Ophthalmic artery
    B. Carotico-tympanic artery
    C. Anterior cerebral artery
    D. Posterior cerebral artery
    E. Anterior choroidal artery

Ans.   40. B   41. A   42. D   43. C   44. D   45. A   46. D

47. **The infraorbital artery is the branch of**
    A. facial artery
    B. ophthalmic artery
    C. maxillary artery
    D. superficial temporal artery
    E. none of the above arteries

48. **The deep cervical artery is the branch of**
    A. inferior thyroid artery
    B. vertebral artery
    C. thyrocervical trunk
    D. costocervical trunk
    E. none of the above arteries

49. **The facial artery terminates by anastomosing with the**
    A. facial artery of the opposite side
    B. infraorbital artery
    C. dorsal nasal branch of ophthalmic artery
    D. transverse facial artery
    E. none of the above arteries

50. **The main tonsillar artery is the branch of the**
    A. ascending palatine artery
    B. ascending pharyngeal artery
    C. lingual artery
    D. facial artery
    E. greater palatine artery

51. **Brachial plexus roots emerge between**
    A. sternomastoid and scalenus anterior
    B. scalenus anterior and scalenus medius
    C. scalenus medius and scalenus posterior
    D. scalenus medius and levator scapulae

52. **Which of the following nerves does *not* contribute to the formation of ansa cervicalis?**
    A. C1
    B. C2
    C. C3
    D. C4

Ans.   47. C   48. D   49. C   50. D   51. B   52. D

53. **Accessory nerve leaves the cranium through which foramen?**
    A. Foramen magnum
    B. Jugular foramen
    C. Posterior condylar canal
    D. Anterior condylar canal

54. **Facial nerve supplies all the following muscles** *except*
    A. fronto-occipitalis
    B. orbicularis occuli
    C. buccinator
    D. masseter

55. **Which of the following muscles is supplied by facial nerve?**
    A. Stylohyoid
    B. Styloglossus
    C. Stylopharyngeus
    D. Anterior belly of digastric

56. **Which of the following muscles is *not* supplied by ansa cervicalis?**
    A. Sternothyroid
    B. Thyrohyoid
    C. Sternohyoid
    D. Omohyoid

57. **The glossopharyngeal nerve supplies**
    A. superior constrictor of pharynx
    B. palatopharyngeus
    C. stylopharyngeus
    D. styloglossus
    E. stylohyoid

58. **Which of the following muscles in *not* supplied by the vago-accessory complex?**
    A. Tensor palati
    B. Palatoglossus
    C. Palatopharyngeus
    D. Constrictors of pharynx

Ans. 53. B   54. D   55. A   56. B   57. C   58. A

59. Which of the following muscles is supplied by the superior laryngeal nerve or its bran
   A. Posterior cricoarytenoid
   B. Inferior constrictor of pharynx
   C. Thyrohyoid
   D. Lateral cricoarytenoid

60. The recurrent laryngeal nerve supplies the
   A. vocalis
   B. inferior constrictor of pharynx
   C. mucosa of larynx
   D. cricothyroid joint
   E. all the above

61. The oculomotor nerve supplies the
   A. superior oblique
   B. orbicularis oculi
   C. dilator pupillae
   D. inferior rectus
   E. none of the above muscles

62. The muscle supplied by trochlear nerve is
   A. inferior oblique
   B. superior oblique
   C. superior rectus
   D. inferior rectus
   E. none of the above

63. The ophthalmic nerve
   A. passes through the lateral wall of cavernous sinus
   B. carries parasympathetic fibres for sphincter pupillae
   C. carries afferent fibres for light reflex
   D. injury results is ophthalmoplegia
   E. is accompanied by ophthalmic artery

64. The longest cranial nerve in the body is the
   A. trigeminal
   B. oculomotor
   C. facial
   D. vagus

Ans.   59. B   60. E   61. D   62. B   63. A   64. D

65. Which of the following nerves is *not* a branch of the posterior division of mandibular nerve?
    A. Buccal
    B. Auriculotem...
    C. Lingual
    D. Inferior alveolar

66. Which of the following nerves is *not* accompanied by the artery of the same name?
    A. Infraorbital nerve
    B. Lingual nerve
    C. Inferior alveolar nerve
    D. Posterior superior alveolar nerve

67. Pterygopalatine ganglion is a
    A. sensory ganglion
    B. sympathetic ganglion
    C. parasympathetic ganglion
    D. pseudoganglion

68. Which of the following structures is *not* supplied by fibres of hypoglossal nerve?
    A. Genioglossus
    B. Geniohyoid
    C. Superior longitudinal muscle of tongue
    D. Hyoglossus

69. The afferent fibres to carotid sinus come from
    A. glossopharyngeal nerve
    B. vagus nerve
    C. sympathetic trunk
    D. all the above nerves

70. Which of the following structures lies just behind the carotid sheath?
    A. Vagus nerve
    B. Superior root of ansa cervicalis
    C. Inferior root of ansa cervicalis
    D. Sympathetic trunk

Ans. 65. A 66. B 67. C 68. B 69. A 70. D

71. **Secretomotor fibres to parotid gland finally reach the gland through**
    A. great auricular nerve
    B. auriculotemporal nerve
    C. tympanic nerve
    D. chorda tympani

72. **Lingual nerve carries all the following fibres *except***
    A. taste fibres from anterior 2/3 of tongue
    B. pain fibres from tongue
    C. secretomotor fibres for sublingual gland
    D. motor fibres for intrinsic muscles of tongue

73. **Which of the following does *not* form part of secretomotor pathway for lacrimal gland?**
    A. Facial nerve
    B. Nerve of pterygoid canal
    C. Otic ganglion
    D. Zygomatic nerve

74. **In relation to lacrimal gland, all the following statements are true *except***
    A. ducts of orbital part drain through palpebral part.
    B. orbital and palpebral parts are continuous.
    C. removal of orbital part is equivalent to functional removal of the whole gland.
    D. removal of the whole of lacrimal gland will not make the conjunctiva dry.

75. **Which of the following structures is *not* present in posterior triangle?**
    A. Suprascapular nerve
    B. Occipital artery
    C. Brachial plexus
    D. Deep cervical lymph nodes

76. **Which of the following structures does *not* form part of eyelid?**
    A. Tarsal plate
    B. Meibomian glands
    C. Orbital septum
    D. Ciliaris muscle

Ans.   71. B   72. D   73. C   74. C   75. D   76. D

77. **Superior ophthalmic vein communicates directly with all the following** *except*
    A. cavernous sinus
    B. angular vein
    C. pterygoid venous plexus
    D. inferior ophthalmic vein

78. **Tears pass through all the following structures** *except*
    A. conjunctival sac
    B. lacrimal sac
    C. frontonasal duct
    D. inferior meatus of nose

79. **Lacrimal gland drains into superior fornix by**
    A. one duct
    B. two ducts
    C. three ducts
    D. many ducts

80. **Which of the following muscles does** *not* **contract for near vision?**
    A. Ciliaris
    B. Dilator pupillae
    C. Medial rectus
    D. Levator palpabrae superioris

81. **The maximum concentration of cones is at the**
    A. optic disc
    B. macula lutea
    C. fovea centralis
    D. ora serrata

82. **The ciliary muscle**
    A. is supplied by parasympathetic nerves
    B. is part of the fibrous coat of eyeball
    C. affects size of pupil
    D. on contraction makes the lens less convex

83. **Medial check ligament**
    A. is the thickened part of orbital periosteum
    B. is part of fascial sheath of medial rectus muscle

Ans. 77. C   78. C   79. D   80. B   81. C   82. A

    C. is part of fascial sheath of superior oblique muscle

    D. checks medial movement of eyeball

84. Constriction of pupil occurs

    A. due to the contraction of ciliary muscle

    B. due to the overactivity of sympathetic nerves

    C. only during light reflex

    D. during light and accommodation reflex

85. Which of the following nerves does *not* supply the tympanic membrane?

    A. Vagus

    B. Glossopharyngeal

    C. Facial

    D. Mandibular

86. Which of the following arteries does *not* supply the middle ear?

    A. Anterior tympanic artery

    B. Deep auricular artery

    C. Stylomastoid artery

    D. Carotico-tympanic artery

87. On which wall of middle ear the pharyngotympanic tube opens?

    A. Anterior

    B. Posterior

    C. Lateral

    D. Medial

88. Which of the following is *not* a part of bony labyrinth?

    A. Modiolus

    B. Vestibule

    C. Promontory

    D. Semicircular duct

89. Fenestra vestibuli is closed by the

    A. secondary tympanic membrane

    B. vestibular membrane

    C. head of stapes

    D. head of malleus

    E. none of the above

Ans.   83. B   84. D   85. C   86. B   87. A   88. D   89. E

90. **The cochlear ganglion lies**
    A. on vestibular membrane
    B. in spiral lamina
    C. just deep to internal acoustic meatus
    D. in the organ of Corti
    E. none of the above

91. **Which of the following is *not* a part of membranous labyrinth?**
    A. Utricle
    B. Ampullary crest
    C. Otoliths
    D. Perilymph
    E. Cochlear duct

92. **Which of the following paranasal sinuses opens in the hiatus semilunaris?**
    A. Sphenoidal sinus
    B. Middle ethmoidal sinuses
    C. Maxillary sinus
    D. All of the above
    E. None of the above

93. **In the erect posture, gravity does *not* favour the drainage of**
    A. frontal sinus
    B. ethmoidal sinus
    C. sphenoidal sinus
    D. maxillary sinus

94. **The most anterior part of nasal septum is formed by the**
    A. vomer
    B. ethmoid
    C. septal cartilage
    D. greater alar cartilage
    E. none of the above

95. **The tubal orifice in the lateral wall of the nasopharynx lies at the level of**
    A. superior nasal concha
    B. middle nasal concha
    C. inferior nasal concha
    D. floor of nasal cavity

Ans.   90. B   91. D   92. C   93. D   94. D   95. C

96. **The palatine tonsil is related laterally to all the following structures** *except*
    A. superior constrictor
    B. palatopharyngeus
    C. prevertebral fascia
    D. pharyngobasilar fascia
    E. glossopharyngeal nerve

97. **The palatine tonsil generally involutes after the age of**
    A. 3 years
    B. 7 years
    C. 14 years
    D. 40 years

98. **At the level of upper border of thyroid cartilage**
    A. pharynx terminates and esophagus begins
    B. the common carotid artery bifurcates
    C. rima glottidis is present
    D. lower border of sixth cervical vertebra is present

99. **Which of the following structures passes deep to the lower border of inferior constrictor muscle of pharynx?**
    A. Recurrent laryngeal nerve and inferior thyroid artery
    B. Recurrent laryngeal nerve and inferior laryngeal artery
    C. Internal laryngeal nerve and superior laryngeal artery
    D. Internal laryngeal nerve and inferior laryngeal artery

100. **The piriform recess is present**
    A. behind the tubal orifice in the nasopharynx
    B. between median and lateral glosso-epiglottic folds in the oropharynx
    C. between thyrohyoid membrane and aryepiglottic fold in the laryngopharynx
    D. between the two vestibular folds in larynx
    E. between nasal notches of the two maxillae

101. **The laryngopharynx has all the following features,** *except*
    A. communicates with larynx through rima glottidis
    B. has piriform recess on either side
    C. ends at the level of C6 vertebra
    D. receives sensory innervation from internal laryngeal nerve

Ans.   96. C   97. C   98. B   99. B   100. C   101. A

102. **All the following features pertain to parathyroid glands
     *except***
     A. they are two in number, superior and inferior parathyroids
     B. each gland is about 0.5 cm in size, yellowish brown in colour
     C. superior parathyroid is more constant in position
     D. inferior parathyroid may rarely be located in superior
        mediastinum

103. **Which of the following structures is *not* related to posterior
     aspect of thyroid gland?**
     A. Internal carotid artery
     B. Internal jugular vein
     C. Parathyroid gland
     D. Vagus nerve

104. **The lateral to medial relationship of facial nerve, external
     carotid artery and retromandibular vein, as they pass through
     parotid gland, is**
     A. nerve, artery, vein
     B. nerve, vein, artery
     C. vein, artery, nerve
     D. vein, nerve, artery

105. **The parotid duct opens**
     A. in the vestibule of mouth opposite upper second molar tooth
     B. in the vestibule of mouth opposite upper second premolar tooth
     C. in the oral cavity opposite upper second molar tooth
     D. in the floor of the mouth on either side of frenulum of tongue

106. **Which of the following structures is not traversing the
     infratemporal fossa?**
     A. Maxillary nerve
     B. Mandibular nerve
     C. Lingual nerve
     D. Lingual artery
     E. Inferior alveolar artery

107. **Which of the following does *not* communicate directly with
     pterygoid venous plexus?**
     A. Maxillary vein
     B. Deep facial vein

Ans.   102. A   103. A   104. B   105. A   106. D   107. C

C. Cavernous sinus

D. Inferior ophthalmic vein

108. **Which of the following actions is the prime action of the muscle which is inserted into coronoid process?**
   A. Depression of mandible
   B. Elevation of mandible
   C. Protraction of mandible
   D. Side to side movement of mandible

109. **Which of the following actions is the prime action of the muscle arising from medial surface of lateral pterygoid plate?**
   A. Elevation of mandible
   B. Retraction of mandible
   C. Elevation of soft palate
   D. Tense the soft palate

110. **Which of the following statements pertaining to sulcus terminalis of tongue is *not* true?**
   A. Its apex is directed anteriorly
   B. Circumvallate papillae lie just in front of it
   C. Behind it lie lymphoid nodules under the mucous membrane
   D. It separates developmentally different parts of tongue

111. **Which of the following structures passes deep to hyoglossus muscle?**
   A. Lingual nerve
   B. Glossopharyngeal nerve
   C. Hypoglossal nerve
   D. Submandibular duct

112. **Which of the following structures pierces the sphenomandibular ligament?**
   A. Inferior alveolar nerve
   B. Lingual nerve
   C. Mylohyoid nerve
   D. Auriculotemporal nerve
   E. None of the above

113. **The articular disc of the temporomandibular joint**
   A. is made up of elastic cartilage
   B. gives attachment to medial pterygoid muscle

Ans.   108. B   109. A   110. A   111. B   112. C

    C. divides the joint cavity into anterior and posterior compartments

    D. is pulled forwards during opening of the jaw

    E. has none of the above characters

114. Which of the following actions is *not* done by the muscle inserted into the articular disc of the temporomandibular joint?

    A. Protraction of mandible

    B. Elevation of mandible

    C. Pull the head of mandible forward

    D. Side to side movement of mandible

115. Which of the following statements is true for the otic ganglion?

    A. It lies on the lateral aspect of the mandibular nerve

    B. It contains postganglionic parasympathetic neurons

    C. It supplies the palatine gland

    D. The nerves to tensor tympani and tensor palati synapse with its neurons

116. The nerve relaying in the pterygopalatine ganglion reaches the ganglion through the

    A. foramen rotundum

    B. sphenopalatine foramen

    C. greater palatine canal

    D. pterygoid canal

    E. inferior orbital fissure

117. Infections from pterygopalatine fossa can travel to

    A. orbital cavity

    B. middle cranial fossa

    C. nasal cavity

    D. oral cavity

    E. all the above

118. The submental lymph nodes drain lymph from all the following areas *except* the

    A. tip of the tongue

    B. median part of the lower lip

    C. median part of the upper lip

    D. chin

    E. median part of the floor of the mouth

Ans. 113. D 114. B 115. B 116. D 117. E 118. C

119. **Which of the following is** *not* **a weak spot and a common site of fracture of mandible?**
    A. Neck
    B. Angle
    C. Body in the region of canine socket
    D. Coronoid process

120. **A fracture through floor of the orbit might result in sensory loss to the**
    A. skin of the forehead
    B. upper eyelid
    C. lower lip
    D. upper incisors and canine teeth

121. **A fracture passing across foramen ovale may result in all the following features** *except*
    A. sensory loss to anterior 2/3 of tongue
    B. sensory loss to lower molars
    C. sensory loss to upper lip
    D. paralysis of tensor palati muscle

122. **All the following features emphasise the clinical importance of fontanelles in the neonate** *except*
    A. they prevent overlapping of bones during childbirth.
    B. state of hydration can be judged.
    C. intracranial pressure can be judged.
    D. they allow growth of brain after birth.

123. **Which nerve is likely to be injured while ligating superior thyroid artery?**
    A. Vagus
    B. Superior laryngeal
    C. External laryngeal
    D. Recurrent laryngeal

124. **All the following features pertain to parotid swellings** *except*
    A. swellings are very painful due to the unyielding nature of parotid fascia.
    B. swelling often pushes the ear lobule upwards.
    C. parotid abscess should be drained by vertical incision.
    D. pain is relieved after taking meals as the secretions get drained.

Ans.   119. D   120. D   121. C   122. A   123. C   124. C

125. **Ulcer on tongue with involvement of lingual nerve can give rise to referred pain in the ear due to which of the following nerves?**
   A. Tympanic nerve
   B. Posterior auricular nerve
   C. Auriculotemporal nerve
   D. Great auricular nerve

126. **A person is unable to suck liquids through a straw. This may be due to lesion of**
   A. mandibular nerve
   B. lingual nerve
   C. glossopharyngeal nerve
   D. facial nerve

127. **Large goitre can produce all the following symptoms *except***
   A. dyspnoea
   B. dysarthria
   C. dysphagia
   D. dysphonia

128. **Bleeding during tonsillectomy usually comes from which of the following vessels?**
   A. Internal jugular vein
   B. Internal carotid artery
   C. Paratonsillar vein
   D. Facial artery

129. **Which of the following arteries does *not* participate in formation of anastomosis in Little's area?**
   A. Superior labial
   B. Lesser palatine
   C. Sphenopalatine
   D. Anterior ethmoidal

130. **During otoscopic examination of tympanic membrane the cone of light is seen in which of the following quadrants?**
   A. Posterosuperior
   B. Anterosuperior
   C. Posteroinferior
   D. Anteroinferior

Ans.   125. C 126. D 127. B 128. C 129. B 130. D

131. A tumor invading jugular foramen may lead to all the following features *except*
   A. loss of hearing
   B. loss of taste sensation from posterior 1/3rd of tongue
   C. increased intracranial pressure
   D. paralysis of muscles of soft palate

132. Injury to oculomotor nerve will produce all the following effects *except*
   A. dilatation of pupil
   B. ptosis
   C. medial squint
   D. loss of accommodation

133. Injury to trigeminal nerve may result in loss of all following reflexes *except*
   A. corneal reflex
   B. sneeze reflex
   C. gag reflex
   D. jaw jerk reflex

134. The 'Surgical flaps of the scalp' during craniotomy comprise first 3 layers of scalp and flaps are turned downwards and not upwards. All the following features explain this statement *except*
   A. these three layers are united intimately by dense connective tissue.
   B. these are separated from pericranium by loose connective tissue.
   C. main arteries and nerves lie deep to these three layers.
   D. nerves and vessels enter the scalp from periphery.

135. Which of the following is called anaesthetist's artery because of being often used for measuring pulse by anaesthetist?
   A. Deep temporal
   B. Superficial temporal
   C. Supraorbital
   D. Infraorbital

Ans.   131. A   132. C   133. C   134. C   135. B

136. 'Dangeous area of face' includes all the following *except*
   A. upper lip
   B. lower lip
   C. lower part of nose
   D. medial part of cheek

137. Which of the following features will distinguish whether injury of facial nerve is at stylomastoid foramen or in upper part of facial canal?
   A. Dribbling of saliva.
   B. Inability to inflate cheek properly.
   C. Loss of taste sensation from anterior 2/3rd of tongue.
   D. Inability to close the eye.

138. Enlargement of hypophysis cerebri can result in all the following features *except*
   A. homonymous hemianopsia
   B. ocular palsy
   C. papillaedema
   D. inability to close the eyes

139. All the following statements regarding cervical part of esophagus are true *except*
   A. it is 5-6 cm long
   B. more easily approachable through right neck incision
   C. lies just anterior to prevertebral fasica
   D. lymphatic drainage is into lower deep cervical lymphnodes

140. All the following statements concerning cervical rib are correct *except*
   A. arises from C7 vertebra
   B. can give rise to a palpable bony lump in the lower part of neck
   C. can cause vascular symptoms due to compression of subclavian artery
   D. can cause compression of seventh cervical nerve

Ans.   136. B   137. C   138. D   139. B   140. D

Directions: For each of the incomplete statements or questions below one or more completions or answers given is correct, Select
- A. if only 1,2 and 3 are correct;
- B. if only 1 and 3 are correct;
- C. if only 2 and 4 are correct;
- D. if only 4 is correct;
- E. if all are correct.

141. The sternomastoid muscle
1. tilts the head on the same side
2. overlaps the carotid sheath
3. is supplied by the spinal part of the accessory nerve and ventral rami of second and third cervical nerves
4. can assist in forced inspiration

142. The scalenus medius muscle
1. arises from posterior tubercles of cervical vertebrae
2. is inserted into the scalene tubercle
3. is related anteriorly to the brachial plexus
4. forms the lateral boundary of vertebral triangle

143. The semispinalis capitis muscle
1. lies in the roof of the suboccipital triangle
2. is inserted on the mastoid process deep to longissimus capitis
3. often shows a tendinous intersection
4. turns the face to the same side

144. The infrahyoid muscles are
1. deep to the pretracheal fascia
2. all supplied by ansa cervicalis
3. all arranged in one plane
4. depressors of hyoid bone

145. The medial pterygoid muscle
1. has an upper head which arises from the infratemporal surface of greater wing of sphenoid
2. is supplied by a branch from anterior division of mandibular nerve
3. retracts the mandible
4. alongwith lateral pterygoid muscle produces side to side chewing movements

Ans.   141. E   142. B   143. B   144. D   145. D

146. **The internal carotid artery**
1. begins at the upper border of cricoid cartilage
2. enters the skull through the carotid canal
3. is separated from the external carotid artery by the posterior belly of digastric muscle
4. lies medial to the internal jugular vein in the carotid sheath

147. **The external cartoid artery**
1. terminates behind the neck of mandible by dividing into maxillary and posterior auricular arteries
2. is contained within the carotid sheath
3. shows a dilatation called carotid sinus at its proximal end
4. is separated from the internal carotid artery by styloid process and structures attached to it

148. **Ligation of external caroid artery just above the level of the tip of the greater cornu is likely to affect the blood flow through**
1. infraorbital artery
2. supraorbital artery
3. transverse facial artery
4. dorsal lingual artery

149. **Which of the following statements are true about the carotid body and carotid sinus?**
1. They lie at the bufurcation of the common carotid artery
2. The carotid sinus contains chemoreceptors
3. The carotid body affects the rate of respiration
4. The carotid sinus affects the blood pressure and the rate of respiration.

150. **The right common carotid artery**
1. is a branch of the arch of aorta
2. passes through the vertebral triangle
3. can be compressed against the carotid tubercle of fifth cervical vertebra
4. runs lateral to the trachea

Ans. 146. C 147. D 148. B 149. B 150. C

151. **The internal jugular vein**
    1. begins as the continuation of the transverse sinus
    2. terminates by joining subclavian vein to form superior vena cava
    3. is accompanied by VII, IX and X cranial nerves as it exits the skull
    4. lies lateral to the common carotid and internal carotid arteries

152. **The middle meningeal artery**
    1. is a branch of second part of maxillary artery
    2. enters the skull through foramen ovale
    3. runs is subdural space
    4. does not supply arachnoid and pia mater

153. **The subclavian vein**
    1. lies anterio-inferior to the subclavian artery
    2. receives entire blood from the upper limb
    3. receives part of the blood from head and neck
    4. receives part of the blood from spinal cord through the vertebral vein

154. **The facial artery**
    1. arises from the external carotid artery just above the tip of the greater cornu of the hyoid bone
    2. enters the face at the postero-inferior angle of the masseter muscle
    3. terminates by anastomosing with a branch of ophthalmic artery
    4. gives tonsillar and ascending pharyngeal arteries

155. **The central artery of retina**
    1. is a branch of ophthalmic artery
    2. runs through the substance of optic nerve
    3. is an end artery
    4. can be examined in a living individual

156. **The ophthalmic artery**
    1. is a branch of internal carotid artery
    2. enters the orbit through superior orbital fissure
    3. establishes anastomosis between internal carotid and external carotid arteries
    4. gives branches to all parts of the eyeball

Ans.   151. D 152. D 153. A 154. B 155. E 156. B

157. **The lingual artery**
    1. arises above the level of hyoid bone
    2. passes superficial to hyoglossus muscle
    3. when ligated, ipsilateral half of the tongue will undergo nerosis
    4. is crossed by hypoglossal nerve

158. **The internal jugular vein**
    1. shows a dilatation in its middle
    2. is overlapped throughout by sternomastoid
    3. receives all veins from thyroid gland
    4. is surrounded by the deep cervical lymph nodes

159. **The vertebral artery**
    1. is a branch of first part of subclavian artery
    2. enters the foramen transversarium of seventh cervical vertebra
    3. runs backwards and medially after coming out of the foramen transversarium of atlas vertebra
    4. runs in the subdural space in its intracranial course

160. **The vertebral vein**
    1. begins at the lower border of pons
    2. comes out of the foramen transversarium of the sixth cervical vertebra
    3. terminates in the subclavian vein
    4. communicates with the internal and external vertebral venous plexuses

161. **The right subclavian artery**
    1. is the branch of the brachiocephalic trunk
    2. arches in front of cervical pleura
    3. can be compressed by cervical rib
    4. terminates at the inner border of first rib to become axillary artery

162. **The left subclavian artery**
    1. is the first branch of the arch of aorta
    2. lies anterior to the scalenus anterior which separates it from the subclavian vein behind
    3. gives dorsal scapular artery from its first part
    4. is related to brachial plexus in its third part

Ans. 157. D 158. C 159. B 160. C 161. A 162. D

163. **The glossopharyngeal nerve**
    1. supplies all muscles of tongue except palatoglossus
    2. is attached to medulla oblongata between the olive and the inferior cerebellar peduncle
    3. supplies taste fibres to epiglottis and vallecula
    4. passes through jugular foramen

164. **The glossopharyngeal nerve**
    1. supplies middle ear
    2. contains secretomotor fibres for the parotid gland
    3. passes deep to posterior border of hyglossus muscle
    4. supplies palatine tonsil

165. **The vagus nerve**
    1. is attached to medulla oblongata between pyramid and olive
    2. is joined by accessory nerve in the jugular foramen
    3. has three ganglia
    4. lies between the internal jugular vein and internal carotid artery within the carotid sheath

166. **The vagus nerve supplies**
    1. dura mater of posterior cranial fossa
    2. taste buds in the region of vallecula
    3. all muscle of larynx
    4. all muscles of pharynx

167. **The spinal part of accessory nerve**
    1. fibres leave the spinal cord through ventral roots of upper five cervical nerves
    2. enters the skull through foramen magnum
    3. runs through the floor of the posterior triangle of neck
    4. supplies the sternomastoid and the trapezius muscles only

168. **The hypoglossal nerve**
    1. supplies only extrinsic muscles of tongue
    2. carries sensory fibres from the inferior surface of tongue
    3. passes deep to the hyglossus muscle
    4. injury results in difficulty in swallowing

Ans.   163. C 164. E 165. C 166. A 167. C 168. D

169. **The left recurrent laryngeal nerve**
    1. winds round the arch of aorta anterior to the ligamentum arteriosum
    2. ascends in the groove between trachea and esophagus
    3. is closely related to the superior thyroid artery
    4. enters the larynx just behind the cricothyroid joint

170. **The facial nerve**
    1. is attached at the lower border of pons just superolateral to the pyramid
    2. leaves the cranial cavity through the internal acoustic meatus
    3. supplies both bellies of the digastric and the stylohyoid muscles in neck
    4. supplies all muscles of facial expression

171. **The optic nerve**
    1. leaves the orbit through optic canal
    2. is surrounded by an extension of subarachnoid space
    3. enters the eyeball 3 mm to the nasal side of the posterior pole of eyeball
    4. carries all visual impulses to the brain

172. **The oculomotor nerve**
    1. arises in the midbrain
    2. runs through the cavernous sinus inferolateral to the internal carotid artery
    3. enters the orbit through the superior orbital fissure
    4. injury results in constriction of pupil

173. **The abducent nerve**
    1. is attached to the upper border of pons
    2. runs through the lateral wall of the cavernous sinus
    3. enters the orbit through the inferior orbital fissure
    4. supplies only lateral rectus muscle

174. **The olfactory nerves**
    1. are about 15-20 in number
    2. carry the sense of smell, from the entire nasal mucosa
    3. pass through the cribriform plate of ethmoid
    4. are formed by the axons of neurons of olfactory bulb

Ans.   169. C 170. C 171. E 172. B 173. D 174. B

175. **The ophthalmic nerve (or its branches)**
    1. runs through the lateral wall of the cavernous sinus
    2. enter the orbit through the superior orbital fissure
    3. carriers afferents for corneal reflex
    4. injury results in diplopia

176. **The mandibular nerve**
    1. leaves the cranial cavity through foramen rotundum
    2. is functionally related to the otic ganglion
    3. runs through the mandibular canal
    4. supplies all the four muscles of mastication

177. **The posterior superior alveolar nerve**
    1. is a branch of the mandibular nerve
    2. runs on the posterior surface of maxilla
    3. supplies the soft palate
    4. supplies the maxillary air sinus and the upper molars

178. **The lingual nerve**
    1. is a branch of the anterior division of mandibular nerve
    2. enters the tongue deep to hyoglossus muscle
    3. is sensory only to the tongue
    4. can be easily anaesthetised where it lies just medial to the
       lower last molar tooth

179. **The inferior cervical ganglion**
    1. is connected to the lower four cervical nerves by the grey rami
       communicantes
    2. receives white ramus communicans from the first thoracic nerve
    3. is connected to the superior cervical ganglion by the ansa
       subclavia
    4. gives plexuses around vertebral and subclavian arteries

180. **The features of Horner's syndrome include**
    1. dilation of pupil
    2. ptosis
    3. increased sweating on face
    4. flushing of face

181. **In relation to eyeball**
    1. in the anatomical position visual axis lies parallel to the orbital
       axis

Ans.   175. A 176. D 177. C 178. D 179. D 180. C

2. the posterior chamber lies behind the lens
3. the fovea centralis is a depression in the center of the optic disc
4. the choroid is the vascular layer

182. **Which of the following statements is/are true for the aqueous humour?**
1. It is present both in the anterior and posterior chambers
2. It is produced by the ciliary muscle
3. It is drained through the irido-corneal angle which lies between the sclera and the iris
4. Its pressure falls in a condition called glucoma

183. **The cornea**
1. is the transparent anterior part of the eyeball
2. has no role in the refraction of the light rays
3. is richly supplied by nerves
4. is supplied by ciliary arteries

184. **Which of the following statements is/are true in relation to the retina?**
1. It is the light sensitive layer
2. Maximum number of cones are present in the region of the optic disc
3. The nervous layer stops at the ora serrata
4. Forms suspensory ligament of lens anteriorly

185. **All the recti muscles of the eyeball**
1. take origin from the common tendinous ring
2. are inserted in front of the equator of the eyeball
3. pierce the fascia bulbi
4. are supplied by the oculomotor nerve

186. **The inferior oblique muscle**
1. arises from the maxilla in the floor of the orbit
2. is inserted 5-6 mm behind the sclero-corneal junction
3. produces elevation, abduction and extortion of eyeball
4. is supplied by the trochlear nerve

187. **The external auditory meatus**
1. is bony in its medial 1/3 part
2. is narrowest at the junction of its bony and cartilaginous parts

---

Ans.   181. D 182. B 183. B 184. B 185. A 186. B

3. is a straight passage
4. is supplied by the fifth and tenth nerves

188. The tympanic membrane
1. is flaccid in most of its extent
2. is convex towards the middle ear
3. has handle of malleus and long process of incus embedded in it
4. is related to the chorda tympani nerve in its upper part

189. The tympanic cavity
1. is narrowest near its floor
2. communicates with the mastoid antrum anteriorly
3. communicates with the internal ear through fenestra vestibuli
4. is supplied by the glossopharyngeal nerve

190. The utricle
1. is the part of membranous labyrinth which lies in the vestibule
2. is concerned with equillibrium
3. is filled with endolymph
4. can be examined by the auroscope

191. The organ of Corti
1. lies on the basilar membrane
2. is concerned with hearing
3. is innervated by the peripheral processes of cells of cochlear ganglion
4. is surrounded by perilymph

192. In relation to the superior constrictor of pharynx
1. its upper border is throughout attached to the skull
2. its lower border overlaps the middle constrictor muscle
3. it takes origin from pharygeal raphe
4. it is pierced by the tonsillar artery

193. The features seen on the lateral wall of the nasopharynx include
1. tubal elevation
2. pharyngeal recess
3. salpingopharyngeal fold
4. nasopharyngeal tonsil

Ans.   187. D 188. C 189. D 190. A 191. A 192. D 193. A

194. **The palatine tonsil**
    1. lies between palatopharyngeal and palatoglossal folds
    2. is made up of lymphoid tissue and mucous glands
    3. is supplied by glossopharyngeal nerve
    4. is mainly supplied by the maxillary artery

195. **Which of the following statements is/are true for larynx?**
    1. It lies opposite the 2nd to 6th cervical vertebrae
    2. It communicates with the pharynx anteriorly
    3. The inlet of larynx is closed by adduction of the vocal cords
    4. The laryngeal prominence is part of the thyroid cartilage

196. **Which of the following statements is/are true about larynx?**
    1. Sensory supply is by recurrent laryngeal nerve only
    2. Intrinsic muscles are supplied by branches of vagus nerve
    3. Dose not move with deglutition
    4. Its interior can be examined with a laryngoscope

197. **The thyroid gland**
    1. moves up and down with deglutition
    2. is drained by veins which accompany the corresponding arteries
    3. enlargement may be associated with hypo or hyper functioning of the gland
    4. surgery may lead to injury to recurrent laryngeal nerve if the inferior thyroid artery is ligated away from the thyroid gland

198. **The thyroid gland**
    1. is enclosed in the pretracheal fascia
    2. has a venous plexus between its true and false capsules
    3. extends superiorly upto the oblique line of the thyroid cartilage
    4. has an isthmus which lies in front of the cricoid cartilage

199. **The parathyroid glands**
    1. are usually two in number
    2. always lie outside the pretracheal fascia
    3. secrete calcitonin
    4. are mainly supplied by the inferior thyroid artery

200. **The parotid gland**
    1. is related superiorly to the external auditory meatus
    2. lies deep to the masseter muscle

Ans.   194. B   195. D   196. C   197. B   198. B   199. D

3. is supplied by secretomotor fibres coming through the
    auriculotemporal nerve
4. is traversed by the facial nerve and facial artery

201. The submandibular salivary gland is
1. completely superficial to the mylohyoid muscle
2. separated from the parotid gland by the stylomandibular
    ligament
3. supplied by secretomotor fibres coming through mandibular
    nerve
4. drained by a single duct which opens under the tongue

202. The lacrimal gland
1. lies in the lacrimal fossa situated at the anteromedial part of
    the roof of the orbit
2. ducts open in the superior fornix of conjunctiva
3. receives its secretomotor nerve supply through the ciliary
    ganglion
4. secretions are meant to keep the cornea moist

**203. Fracture of the base of skull involving foramen ovale is likely
to result in**
1. paralysis of tensor tympani
2. paralysis of anterior belly of digastric
3. loss of exteroceptive sensations from anterior 2/3 of tongue
4. loss of taste sensation from anterior 2/3 of tongue

204. The dorsum of the tongue behind the sulcus terminalis has
1. filliform papillae
2. taste buds
3. vallate papillae
4. lymphoid nodules

**205. Which of the following structures lie just under the mucous
membrane of the floor of mouth (between the mandible and
the tongue)?**
1. Lingual nerve
2. Hypoglossal nerve
3. Submandibular duct
4. Submandibular gland

Ans.   200. B   201. C   202. C   203. A   204. C   205. B

Directions: Each of the following questions consists of an assertion and a reason. Answers should be choosen as follows:
- A. if the assertion and reason are true statements and the reason is a correct explanation of the assertion;
- B. if the assertion and reason are true statements but the reason is not a correct explanation of the assertion;
- C. if the assertion is true but the reason is a false statement;
- D. if the assertion is false but the reason is a true statement;
- E. if both assertion and reason are false statements.

206. **The transverse diameter of the atlas vertebra is the largest of all the cervical vertebrae**
Because
It has no body

207. **Rotation of the vertebral column is free in the lumbar region**
Because
the intervertebral discs are very thin in this region

208. **Only flexion and extension can take place between atlas and axis vertebrae**
Because
rotation between these vertebrae is limited by alar ligaments

209. **The temporomandibular joint is a cartilaginous joint**
Because
it contains an articular disc made of fibrocartilage

210. **Dislocation of the temporomandibular joint generally occurs when the jaw is fully opened**
Because
the capsule of the joint is thin anteriorly

211. **Rupture of anterior division of middle meningeal artery may lead to hemiplegia on the opposite side**
Because
this artery supplies motor area of cerebral cortex

212. **The internal carotid artery can be compressed against carotid tubercle**
Because
anterior tubercle of the sixth cervical vertebra is a large one .

Ans. 206. B 207. E 208. D 209. D 210. C 211. C 212. D

213. **If the maxillary vein is ligated before it joins the superficial temporal vein, blood form infratemporal fossa cannot reach heart**
Because
veins in the infratemporal fossa have no other communications

214. **Thrombosis of the central artery of retina leads to total blindness of that eye**
Because
this is the only artery supplying the eyeball

215. **A fracture through the roof of the maxillary sinus might result in sensory loss to the upper incisors and canine teeth**
Because
the floor of the sinus is related to these teeth

216. **The maxillary air sinus is the most commonly infected sinus**
Because
it is the largest air sinus

217. **Infection in lower teeth and gums is often associated with pain in the ear**
Because
the head of the mandible is closely related to external auditory meatus

218. **In tonsillitis pain is often felt in the ear**
Because
they are both supplied by the glossopharyngeal nerve

219. **Syringing of the external acoustic meatus for removal of wax can sometimes lead to death**
Because
the auricular branch of vagal gets irritated leading to vagal stimulation of heart

220. **While going up in the aeroplane it is advisable to swallow**
Because
the tubal orifice closes during swallowing

Ans.   213. E 214. C 215. C 216. B 217. B 218. A 219. A 220.C

221. **In unconscious person tongue should be kept pulled out mechanically**
    Because
    this will prevent blocking of airway by the tongue falling back

222. **The facial vein is tortuous**
    Because
    it has to accommodate to the movements of mandible

223. **Swellings of parotid gland are *not* very painful**
    Because
    it is separated from the external ear by tympanic membrane

224. **The middle ear cavity does *not* communicate with atmosphere**
    Because
    it is separated from the external ear by tympanic membrane

225. **Incision in the tympanic membrane should be made in its lower part**
    Because
    its upper part is related to the chorda tympani nerve.

226. **To examine the tympanic membrane by auroscope, the auricle is pulled upwards, backwards and laterally**
    Because
    the tympanic membrane is placed obliquely downwards and medially

227. **In cancer of the tip of the tongue the lymph nodes should be examined on both sides**
    Because
    the tip of the tongue can move on both sides

228. **Swellings of thyroid gland move with degutition**
    Because
    the prevertebral fascia connects the gland to thyroid and cricoid cartilages

---

Ans.   221. A 222. D 223. E 224. D 225. A 226. B 227. B 228.C

229. Injury to the oculomotor nerve leads to lateral squint
Because
lateral rectus is the only extraocular muscle which produces abduction of the eyeball

230. Injury to mandibular nerve will interfere in sucking movement
Because
buccinator which is an important muscle involved in sucking, gets paralysed

231. In case of injury to the left mandibular nerve, the mandible deviates to the left side on opening the mouth
Because
the masseter is paralysed

232. Injury to the lingual nerve above its union with chorda tympani will result in loss of taste sensation from anterior 2/3 of tongue
Because
chorda tympani carries taste sensations from this part of tongue

233. Injury to the facial nerve at stylomastoid foramen will impair formation of tears
Because
the lacrimal gland receives its secretomotor supply through the facial nerve

234. In supranuclear paralysis of facial nerve the person is able to smile normally
Because
lower half of the face is represented bilaterally in the cerebral cortex

235. Injury to the hypoglossal nerve leads to difficulty in swallowing
Because
all the muscles of tongue are paralysed

Ans.   229. C 230. E 231. B 232. D 233. D 234. E 235. C

236. **In case of injury to the right hypoglossal nerve the tongue deviates to the left side on protrusion**
Because
unparalysed left genioglossus muscle protrudes the tongue to the left side

237. **Injury to the inferior cervical ganglion will *not* affect the size of pupil**
Because
the postganglionic fibres for dilator pupillae arise from the superior cervical ganglion

238. **The tumours of hypophysis cerebri can lead to hemianopia**
Because
they can press upon nerves passing through the cavernous sinus

239. **In the living individual, vocal cords appear pinkish in colour**
Because
they have many blood vessels in the submucosa

240. **Superior oblique muscle passes superior to the eyeball still it moves the eyeball downwards**
Because
its tendon changes its direction at the trochlea

Ans.   236. E   237. D   238. B   239. E   240. B

CHAPTER 2

The Upper Limb

Directions: Each of the incomplete statements or questions below is followed by four or five suggested completions or answers. Select the one which is BEST in each case.

1. **Which of the following bones develops by intramembranous ossification?**
    - A. Scapula
    - B. Clavicle
    - C. Humerus
    - D. Ulna
    - E. None of the above

2. **Rhomboid fossa is present on**
    - A. the inferior surface of the calvicle
    - B. the root of the spine of the scapula
    - C. the anterior aspect of the lower end of humerus
    - D. the posterior aspect of the lower end of humerus

3. **In relation to scapula**
    - A. the spine is subcutaneous
    - B. inferior angle lies at the level of sixth thoracic vertebra
    - C. lateral border is the thinnest border
    - D. scapular notch transmits suprascapular vessels
    - E. coracoid process can be felt in supraclavicular fossa

4. **The humerus presents**
    - A. medial epicondyle which is smaller than the lateral epicondyle
    - B. coronoid fossa on the posterior aspect of its lower end
    - C. trochlea with a larger lateral flange
    - D. intertubercular sulcus on the medial side
    - E. anatomical neck which is completely intracapsular

Ans.   1. B   2. A   3. A   4. E

5. **In relation to ulna**
   A. it is shorter than the radius
   B. it is the main bone which transmits forces from the hand
   C. its head articulates with the capitulum of humerus
   D. posterior border is subcutaneous
   E. gives insertion to pronator quadratus

6. **In relation to radius**
   A. head articulates with the lateral epicondyle of humerus and the radial notch of ulna
   B. its styloid process lies at a higher level than the styloid process of ulna
   C. shaft is convex laterally
   D. does not give attachment to any of the superficial flexor muscles of forearm
   E. has none of the above properties

7. **The clavicle**
   A. is seldom fractured
   B. is the first bone to ossify in the body
   C. contains a large medullary cavity
   D. laterally articulates with the coracoid process
   E. has conoid tubercle on the sternal end

8. **The following carpal bones lie in the proximal row** *except*
   A. scaphoid
   B. lunate
   C. capitate
   D. triquetral
   E. pisiform

9. **The first metacarpal bone**
   A. articulates proximally with trapezoid
   B. has a secondary ossification centre for its base
   C. lies in the plane of other metacarpal bones
   D. gives attachment to abductor pollicis longus and brevis
   E. forms a saddle joint distally with proximal phalanx

10. **Which metacarpal articulates with three carpal bones?**

A. I	B. II
C. III	D. IV
E. V	

Ans.   5. D   6. C   7. B   8. C   9. B   10. B

11. **The infraglenoid tubercle**
    A. lies about 3 cm. below the glenoid cavity
    B. gives attachment to the long head of biceps brachii
    C. gives attachment to the lateral head of triceps brachii
    D. is intracapsular
    E. has none of the above properties

12. **Which of the following bones has two primary centres of ossification?**
    A. Rib
    B. Clavicle
    C. Fibula
    D. Femur

13. **Which of the following structures passes through the suprascapular notch?**
    A. Subscapular artery
    B. Circumflex scapular artery
    C. Suprascapular nerve
    D. Dorsal scapular nerve

14. **The mammary gland**
    A. consists of 5-10 lobes
    B. lies entirely deep to deep fascia
    C. has an axillary tail
    D. ligaments of Cooper connect it to pectoral fascia.

15. **All the following statements are true for axillary tail of mammary gland** *except*
    A. lies in superficial fascia
    B. lies close to axillary vessels
    C. pierces the deep fascia
    D. it arises from supero-lateral quadrant of mammary gland.

16. **All the following arteries supply the mammary gland** *except*
    A. anterior intercostal arteries
    B. lateral thoracic artery
    C. superior epigastric artery
    D. posterior intercostal arteries

Ans.   11. E   12. B   13. C   14. C   15. A   16. C

17. The posterior wall of axilla consists of all the following muscles *except*
    A. subscapularis
    B. subclavius
    C. latissimus dorsi
    D. teres major

18. The nerve that runs over the medial wall of axilla is
    A. medial pectoral
    B. long thoracic
    C. thoracodorsal
    D. ulnar

19. The axillary lymph nodes drain all the following *except*
    A. upper limb
    B. mammary gland
    C. body wall above the level of umbilicus
    D. side of neck

20. The musculotendinous cuff is formed by all the following muscles *except*
    A. supraspinatus
    B. teres minor
    C. long head of triceps
    D. subscapularis
    E. infraspinatus

21. Which of the following muscles has a double nerve supply?
    A. Biceps brachii
    B. Flexor digitorum superficialis
    C. Flexor digitorum profundus
    D. Coracobrachialis
    E. None of the above

22. Which of the following muscles is a flexor and medial rotator of arm?
    A. Teres major
    B. Pectoralis major
    C. Latissimus dorsi
    D. Coracobrachialis
    E. Subscapularis

Ans. 17. B 18. B 19. D 20. C 21. C 22. B

23. **Which of the following pairs of muscles is the most effective in overhead abduction?**
    A. Trapezius and serratus anterior
    B. Trapezius and deltoid
    C. Serratus anterior and deltoid
    D. Deltoid and supraspinatus

24. **Which of the following muscles is an extensor and lateral rotator of arm?**
    A. Teres major
    B. Latissimus dorsi
    C. Posterior fibres of deltoid
    D. Anterior fibres of deltoid
    E. Sternocostal fibres of pectoralis majoi

25. **Abduction on shoulder joint involves**
    A. glenohumeral joint
    B. sternoclavicular joint
    C. acromioclavicular joint
    D. rotation of scapula
    E. all the above

26. **Which of the following bones does *not* give attachment to triceps?**
    A. Scapula
    B. Humerus
    C. Clavicle
    D. Ulna

27. **Which of the following muscles does not form any boundary of axilla?**
    A. Serratus anterior
    B. Pectoralis major
    C. Subclavius
    D. Subscapularis
    E. Deltoid

28. **Quarangular space is bounded by all the following structures *except* the**
    A. long head of triceps
    B. teres minor

Ans.   23. A   24. C   25. E   26. C   27. E

C. subscapularis
D. infraspinatus
E. surgical neck of humerus

29. Which of the following muscles is *not* a flexor on elbow joint?
A. Biceps brachii
B. Coracobrachialis
C. Brachialis
D. Brachioradialis
E. Pronator teres

30. Which of the following muscles can extend the forearm?
A. Extensor carpi radialis longus
B. Extensor carpi radialis brevis
C. Brachioradialis
D. Anconeus
E. All the above

31. Which of the following muscles is a protractor of scapula?
A. Trapezius
B. Rhomboideus major
C. Pectoralis major
D. Pectoralis minor
E. Deltoid

32. Which of the following muscles does *not* belong to the superficial flexor group of forearm?
A. Pronator teres
B. Flexor carpi radialis
C. Flexor pollicis longus
D. Flexor digitorum superficialis
E. Flexor carpi ulnaris

33. Which of the following structure does *not* pass superficial to flexor retinaculum?
A. Ulnar nerve
B. Ulnar artery
C. Palmaris longus
D. Radial artery
E. Palmar cutaneous branch of median nerve

Ans. 28. D 29. B 30. D 31. D 32. C 33. D

34. **True statement about elbow joint is that**
    A. capsule is thick and strong anteriorly and posteriorly
    B. radial collateral ligament is attached to the head of radius
    C. synovial membrane is pulled up by articularis cubiti during extension
    D. it is a complex joint
    E. it has none of the above properties

35. **Which of the following is *not* a content of cubital fossa?**
    A. Tendon of Biceps brachii
    B. Median nerve
    C. Radial artery
    D. Ulnar artery
    E. Ulnar nerve

36. **Which of the following structures does *not* pass deep to extensor retinaculum?**
    A. Cephalic vein
    B. Posterior interosseous nerve
    C. Anterior interosseous artery
    D. Extensor digiti minimi
    E. Extensor carpi ulnaris   •

37. **Which of the following combination of muscles is best for flexion of wrist?**
    A. Flexor carpi ulnaris and flexor carpi radialis
    B. Flexor carpi ulnaris and flexor digitorum profundus
    C. Flexor carpi radialis and flexor digitorum superficialis
    D. Flexor digitorum profundus and flexor pollicis longus

38. **Which of the following is a prime flexor of meta-carpophalangeal joint?**
    A. Flexor digitorum superficialis
    B. Flexor digitorum profundus
    C. Flexor carpi radialis
    D. Lumbricals
    E. None of the above

39. **Which of the following is a prime flexor of distal inter-phalangeal joint?**
    A. Flexor digitorum superficialis

Ans.   34. E   35. E   36. A   37. A   38. D

B. Flexor digitorum profundus
C. Lumbricals
D. Palmar interossei
E. None of the above

40. The fifth metacarpophalangeal joint
   A. is a hinge joint
   B. has a thick dorsal ligament
   C. is abducted by fourth dorsal interosseous
   D. is extended by extensor digitorum

41. Which of the following is a prime extensor of meta-carpophalangeal joint of thumb?
   A. Extensor pollicis longus
   B. Extensor pollicis brevis
   C. Abductor pollicis longus
   D. First lumbrical
   E. First dorsal interosseous

42. The second lumbrical muscle is supplied by
   A. digital branch of median nerve
   B. superficial branch of ulnar nerve
   C. deep branch of ulnar nerve
   D. both median and ulnar nerve

43. All the muscles on the back of free upper limb are supplied by
   A. median nerve
   B. ulnar nerve
   C. radial nerve
   D. radial and ulnar nerves
   E. radial and median nerves

44. Abduction of thumb occurs on
   A. proximal interphalangeal joint
   B. metacarpophalangeal joint
   C. carpometacarpal joint
   D. intercarpal joint

45. Adductor pollicis is supplied by
   A. median nerve

    B. deep branch of ulnar nerve
    C. superficial branch of ulnar nerve
    D. radial nerve

46. **Which of the following statements is *not* true for adduction of ring finger?**
    A. Ring finger moves laterally in adduction
    B. It involves movement on metacarpophalangeal joint
    C. It is done by palmar interosseous muscle
    D. Median nerve is responsible for it

47. **Hypothenar muscles are supplied by**
    A. ulnar nerve only
    B. median nerve only
    C. median and ulnar nerves
    D. radial nerve only
    E. radial and ulnar nerves

48. **The medial pectoral nerve**
    A. arises from medial cord
    B. pierces the clavipectoral fascia
    C. topographically situated medial to lateral pectoral nerve
    D. supplies pectoralis minor muscle only

49. **The thoracodorsal nerve**
    A. is a branch of lateral cord
    B. is accompanied by a branch of posterior circumflex artery
    C. supplies latissimus dorsi muscle
    D. crosses superficial to axillary vein

50. **The axillary nerve supplies all the following structures *except***
    A. deltoid
    B. teres major
    C. shoulder joint
    D. skin over lower half of deltoid

51. **The long thoracic nerve supplies**
    A. pectoralis minor
    B. teres major
    C. subscapularis
    D. serratus anterior

Ans.   45. B   46. D   47. A   48. A   49. C   50. B   51. D

52. The root value of ulnar nerve is
    A. C5 C6
    B. C6 C7
    C. C7 C8
    D. C8 T1

53. Posterior interosseous nerve passes through which osteofascial compartment under extensor retinaculum?
    A. Second
    B. Third
    C. Fourth
    D. Fifth

54. Which of the following muscles of back is *not* supplied by dorsal rami of spinal nerves?
    A. Rhomboideus major
    B. Erector spinae
    C. Semispinalis capitis
    D. Splenius capitis

55. Which of the following structures does *not* form a content of lower part of anterior compartment of arm?
    A. Median nerve
    B. Radial nerve
    C. Ulnar nerve
    D. Brachial artery

56. Which of the following statements is true about coracobrachialis muscle?
    A. It arises in common with long head of biceps
    B. It is pierced by musculocutaneous nerve
    C. It is inserted into coronoid process of ulna
    D. It is medial rotator of arm

57. All the following features occur at the level of insertion of coracobrachialis muscle *except*
    A. ulnar nerve goes to posterior compartment
    B. radial nerve enters the anterior compartment
    C. median nerve crosses brachial artery
    D. basilic vein becomes axillary vein

Ans.   52. D   53. C   54. A   55. C   56. B   57. D

58. Which of the following statements is *not* true about Flexor digitorum superficialis?
    A. Its synovial sheath is common with that of flexor digitorum profundus
    B. In front of wrist its tendons are arranged in two strata
    C. It is supplied by anterior interosseous nerve
    D. Each of its tendon splits into two before insertion.

59. Which of the following statements is *not* true about Flexor carpi ulnaris?
    A. It is supplied by ulnar nerve
    B. It is inserted into pisiform bone
    C. It flexes the little finger
    D. Pisohamate and pisometacarpal ligaments are continuations of its tendon.

60. Which of the following muscles does *not* help in abduction on wrist joint?
    A. Abductor pollicis longus
    B. Extensor pollicis brevis
    C. Extensor carpi radialis longus
    D. Brachioradialis.

61. Which of the following is *not* a thenar muscle?
    A. Flexor pollicis longus
    B. Opponens pollicis
    C. Abductor pollicis brevis
    D. Flexor pollicis brevis

62. All the following factors add to instability of shoulder joint *except*
    A. shallow glenoid cavity
    B. large head of humerus relative to glenoid cavity
    C. laxity of capsule
    D. intracapsular origin of long head of biceps

63. The labrum glenoidale is
    A. made up of elastic cartilage
    B. triangular in cross section
    C. not covered by synovial membrane
    D. does not add to stability of joint.

Ans.　58. C　59. C　60. D　61. A　62. D　63. B

64. **Which of the following muscles initiates abduction on shoulder joint?**
    A. Supraspinatus
    B. Deltoid
    C. Long head of biceps
    D. Serratus anterior

65. **Which of the following muscles is a flexor of forearm in midprone position?**
    A. Biceps brachii
    B. Brachialis
    C. Brachioradialis
    D. Pronator teres

66. **Which of the following statements regarding carrying angle is true?**
    A. Extended forearm is deviated medially in relation to arm.
    B. It is due to long lateral flange of trochlea
    C. It disappears in prone position
    D. Deviation is less in case of females

67. **Which of the following joints is *not* a hinge joint?**
    A. Elbow
    B. Metacarpophalangeal
    C. Distal Interphalangeal
    D. Proximal Interphalangeal

68. **Which of the following joints has articular disc?**
    A. Metacarpophalangeal
    B. Sternoclavicular
    C. Wrist joint
    D. Superior radioulnar joint

69. **All the following statements are true regarding middle phalanx *except***
    A. dorsally related to extensor apparatus
    B. palmar aspects of its base gives attachment to a slip of palmar aponeurosis
    C. flexor digitorum superficialis is inserted on its base.
    D. flexor digitorum profundus is related to its palmar surface

---

Ans.　64. A　65. C　66. C　67. B　68. B　69. B

70. **Which of the following arteries arises from second part of axillary artery?**
    A. Superior thoracic
    B. Lateral thoracic
    C. Subscapular
    D. Circumflex scapular

71. **Brachial artery lies on the anterior aspect of all the following structures** *except*
    A. teres major
    B. triceps
    C. coracobrachialis
    D. brachialis

72. **All the following are branches of brachial artery** *except*
    A. profunda brachii
    B. nutrient artery to humerus
    C. ulnar collateral
    D. common interosseous

73. **Superficial palmar arch**
    A. lies superficial to palmar aponeurosis
    B. is accompanied by superficial branch of ulnar nerve
    C. gives three common digital arteries
    D. is completed by princeps pollicis artery

74. **In relation to axillary vein, which of the following statements is correct?**
    A. It is the continuation of basilic vein
    B. It pierces the clavipectoral fascia
    C. It terminates into brachiocephalic vein
    D. It lies lateral to the axillary artery

75. **Which of the following arteries accompanies the axillary nerve through the quadrangular space?**
    A. Anterior circumflex humeral artery
    B. Posterior circumflex humeral artery
    C. Circumflex scapular artery
    D. Profunda brachii artery
    E. Suprascapular artery

Ans.   70. B   71. A   72. D   73. C   74. A   75. B

76. **Which of the following is *not* a branch of deep palmar arch?**
    A. Recurrent branches
    B. Perforating arteries
    C. Palmar digital arteries
    D. Palmar metacarpal arteries

77. **Which of the following arteries does not participate in scapular anastomosis?**
    A. Suprascapular
    B. Transverse cervical
    C. Lateral thoracic
    D. Circumflex scapular

78. **Cephalic vein**
    A. arises from the medial end of dorsal venous arch
    B. terminates by joining basilic vein
    C. continues as axillary vein at the lower border of teres major
    D. joins axillary vein in axilla
    E. has none of the above properties

79. **Which of the following muscles will be paralysed when recurrent branch of median nerve is injured?**
    A. Abductor pollicis longus
    B. Extensor pollicis longus
    C. Extensor pollicis brevis
    D. Abductor pollicis brevis
    E. None of the above

80. **Median nerve receives contribution from the**
    A. lateral cord
    B. medial cord
    C. posterior cord
    D. lateral and medial cords
    E. medial and posterior cords

81. **Intercostobrachial nerve is usually a branch of the**
    A. lower trunk of brachial plexus
    B. medial cord
    C. first intercostal nerve
    D. second intercostal nerve
    E. third intercostal nerve

Ans. 76. C 77. C 78. D 79. D 80. D 81. D

82. **The nail bed of middle finger is usually supplied by**
    A. palmar digital branch of ulnar nerve
    B. dorsal branch of ulnar nerve
    C. palmar digital branch of median nerve
    D. radial nerve

83. **The nerve most likely to be injured in fractures of the shaft of the humerus is the**
    A. median
    B. musculocutaneous
    C. radial
    D. axillary
    E. ulnar

84. **The subacromial bursa**
    A. communicates with the synovial cavity of shoulder joint
    B. lies under the tendon of supraspinatus
    C. does not communicate with subdeltoid bursa
    D. lies under the coracoacromial ligament
    E. has all the above properties

85. **The scapula and upper limb are suspended from the clavicle by**
    A. coracoacromial ligament
    B. coracohumeral ligament
    C. coracoclavicular ligament
    D. costoclavicular ligament

86. **Injury to which part of brachial plexus results in "Policeman receiving a tip position" of the upper limb?**
    A. Lateral cord
    B. Upper trunk
    C. Lower trunk
    D. Middle trunk

87. **'Saturday night paralysis' results from injury to**
    A. radial nerve
    B. ulnar nerve
    C. median nerve
    D. musculocutaneous nerve

Ans.   82. C   83. C   84. D   85. C   86. B   87. A

88. **In injury of radial nerve, which of the following movements will *not* be possible?**
    A. Abduction at metacarpophalangeal joints
    B. Adduction at metacarpophalangeal joints
    C. Extension at metacarpophalangeal joints
    D. Extension at interphalangeal joints.

89. **Student's elbow is due to inflammation of**
    A. subcutaneous olecrenon bursa
    B. medial epicondyle
    C. lateral epicondyle
    D. skin over olecrenon

90. **Tennis elbow can result from all the following conditions *except***
    A. sprain of ulnar collateral ligament
    B. tearing of fibres of extensor carpi radialis brevis muscle
    C. inflammation of lateral epicondyle
    D. inflammation of bursa underneath extensor carpi radialis brevis

91. **All the following statements are true regarding fracture of scaphoid *except***
    A. most frequently fractured carpal bone
    B. high incidence of avascular necrosis
    C. low incidence of non-union
    D. clinically diagnosed by tenderness in anatomic snuffbox.

92. **All of the following statements are true about lunate bone *except***
    A. half moon shaped bone
    B. articulates distally with head of capitate
    C. usually dislocates dorsally
    D. median nerve assessment is important in managing its dislocation

93. **All the following statements regarding palmar creases are true *except***
    A. transverse crease in the distal palm corresponds to metacarpophalangeal joints
    B. proximal crease of fingers is located at base of proximal phalanx

Ans.   88. C   89. A   90. A   91. C   92. C

    C. middle crease of fingers is at proximal interphalangeal joint

    D. distal crease of fingers lies opposite distal interphalangeal joint

94. Symptoms of carpal tunnel syndrome pertain to involvement of

    A. flexor digitorum superficialis

    B. flexor digitorum profundus

    C. ulnar nerve

    D. median nerve

95. "Ape" hand deformity results from injury to

    A. ulnar nerve

    B. radial nerve

    C. median nerve

    D. first carpometacarpal joint

96. Sensory loss over lateral half of the anterior surface of forearm is due to involvement of which of the following nerves?

    A. Median

    B. Ulnar

    C. Radial

    D. Musculocutaneous

97. Ulnar bursa communicates distally with digital synovial sheath of which digit?

    A. Little finger

    B. Ring finger

    C. Middle finger

    D. Index finger

98. Fanning of digits is not possible in injury to

    A. radial nerve

    B. deep branch of ulnar nerve

    C. superficial branch of ulnar nerve

    D. median nerve.

99. All the following statements are true about midpalmar space *except*

    A. it lies under medial part of palmar aponeurosis

    B. it communicates with medial three lumbrical canals

    C. it communicates with digital synovial sheaths

    D. it is separated from hypothenar muscles by medial palmar septum

Ans.   93. B   94. D   95. C   96. D   97. A   98. B   99. C

100. The clavicle
   A. articulates with the sternum forming cartilaginous joint
   B. forms a fibrous joint with the acromion
   C. is not united to the clavicle of the opposite side
   D. is convex anteriorly in its medial two third part

Directions: For each of the incomplete statements or questions below, one or more completions or answers given is correct, Select
   A. if only 1,2 and 3 are correct;
   B. if only 1 and 3 are correct;
   C. if only 2 and 4 are correct;
   D. if only 4 is correct;
   E. if all are correct.

---

101. The coracoid process
   1. is subcutaneous
   2. has a bursa underneath it
   3. gives attachment to deltoid
   4. transmits forces from upper limb to the clavicle

102. The fracture of the surgical neck of the humerus is likely to be associated with
   1. paralysis of deltoid muscle
   2. tearing of brachialis muscle
   3. tearing of the capsule of shoulder joint
   4. injury to brachial artery

103. The head of ulna
   1. articulates with ulnar notch of radius
   2. is separated from the wrist joint by an articular disc
   3. is separated from the styloid process by a groove in which lies the tendon of extensor carpi ulnaris
   4. is palpable below the styloid process of ulna

104. The shoulder joint
   1. has a tight capsule
   2. is protected all around by deltoid
   3. communicates with subacromial bursa
   4. allows only about 120° of abduction

Ans.   100. D 101. D 102. B 103. A 104. D

105. The elbow joint
1. is a hinge variety of synovial joint
2. communicates with the superior radioulnar joint
3. is extended primarily by triceps
4. is protected by strong collateral ligaments

106. The superior radioulnar joint
1. is a pivot type of joint
2. is separated from the elbow joint by annular ligament
3. allows movements of supination and pronation
4. is commonly dislocated in adults

107. The wrist joint
1. is formed between ulna, radius, scaphoid, lunate and triquetral
2. is ellipsoid type of synovial joint
3. is flexed primarily by flexor digitorum superficialis and flexor digitorum profundus
4. has greater range of adduction than abduction

108. True statements concering the lunate include
1. it articulates with the articular disc
2. it participates in the midcarpal joint
3. it is usually dislocated anteriorly
4. it articulates with the second metacarpal bone

109. The metacarpophalangeal joint of index finger
1. is a hinge type of synovial joint
2. is flexed by first lumbrical muscle
3. is extended primarily by first dorsal interosseous
4. is abducted by first dorsal interosseous

110. The interosseous membrane
1. has fibres directed upwards and medially
2. gives origin to deep muscles of forearm
3. is pierced by posterior interosseous nerve and artery
4. transmits to ulna force directed upwards from hand and radius

111. The axilla
1. has a posterior wall constituted by scapula and subscapularis muscle
2. has axillary lymph nodes which also drain lymph from the medial part of mammary gland

---

Ans.   105. E   106. B   107. C   108. A   109. C   110. C

3. communicates with neck behind the middle third of clavicle
4. has an anterior wall along which the long thoracic nerve lies

112. The pectoralis major
1. takes origin from the second to sixth ribs
2. is inserted into the lateral lip of bicipital groove
3. is the main adductor and lateral rotator of arm at the shoulder joint
4. is supplied by lateral and medial pectoral nerves

113. The pectoralis minor
1. takes origin from third to fifth ribs
2. is inserted on the tip of acromion process
3. is supplied by medial pectoral nerve
4. protracts the scapula and adducts the arm

114. The serratus anterior
1. is inserted mainly on the superior angle of scapula
2. protracts the scapula and rotates it laterally to produce overhead abduction
3. is supplied by cervical 6,7 and 8 segments of the spinal cord
4. paralysis results in winging of scapula

115. The deltoid muscle
1. takes origin from the posterior border of the lateral third of clavicle
2. is a multipennate muscle
3. is supplied by a branch from lateral cord of brachial plexus
4. produces abduction, flexion and extension on the shoulder joint

116. The biceps brachii
1. has a long head arising from the coracoid process and a short head arising from supraglenoid tubercle of scapula
2. is supplied by median nerve
3. is attached to radius through bicipital aponeurosis
4. is a strong supinator

117. The brachialis
1. is inserted on radial tuberosity
2. has a double nerve supply

Ans.   111. A   112. C   113. B   114. C   115. C   116. D

    3. flexes the arm on shoulder joint

    4. flexes the forearm on elbow joint

118. The triceps muscle

    1. has a long head arising from supraglenoid tubercle of scapula

    2. has a deeper part called articularis cubiti, which is inserted on the capsule of elbow joint

    3. receives all its nerve supply from radial nerve in the radial groove

    4. is the main extensor of forearm

119. The supinator

    1. takes origin from the supinator crest of ulna

    2. is pierced by the posterior intersseous nerve

    3. is a strong supinator when elbow is kept extended

    4. forms the floor of cubital fossa

120. In relations to cubital fossa

    1. the median cubital vein runs obliquely across it

    2. is bounded laterally by the medial border of pronator teres

    3. median nerve leaves the fossa by passing between the two heads of pronator teres

    4. pulsations of brachial artery can be felt just lateral to the tendon of biceps brachii

121. The extensor carpi ulnaris

    1. is supplied by the ulnar nerve

    2. is inserted into the pisiform bone

    3. passes superficial to the extensor retinaculum

    4. produces extension and adduction of hand

122. The flexor carpi radialis

    1. is inserted into the bases of second and third metacarpals

    2. is supplied by radial nerve

    3. has its own synovial sheath

    4. produces flexion of second and third fingers

123. The brachioradialis muscle

    1. takes origin from the lower one third of the lateral supracondylar ridge of humerus

    2. is supplied by the radial nerve

Ans.   117. C 118. C 119. E 120. B 121. D 122. B

3. flexes the hand on the wrist joint
4. brings the forearm in midprone position and flexes it

124. The flexor digitorum profundus
1. is supplied by both ulnar and median nerves
2. tendons are arranged in two layers in front of the wrist joint
3. has a synovial sheath in common with the flexor digitorum superficialis
4. is the prime flexor of proximal interphalangeal joint

125. All the superficial flexor muscles of the forearm
1. arise by a common tendon from the medial epicondyle of humerus
2. are supplied by the median nerve
3. are flexors of the elbow joint
4. enter the hand deep to flexor retinaculum

126. The lumbrical muscles
1. arise from the tendons of flexor digitorum superficialis
2. are supplied by digital branches of ulnar and median nerves
3. pass along the ulnar side of each digit to reach dorsal digital expansion
4. flex the metacarpophalangeal joints and extend the interphalangeal joints

127. The dorsal interossei
1. are bipennate muscles
2. are supplied by the radial nerve
3. are abductors of digits
4. are extensors of metacarpophalangeal joints

128. The thenar space
1. contains thenar muscles
2. is separated from midpalmar space by a septum
3. communicates with the radial bursa
4. is bounded posteriorly by fascia covering the adductor pollicis muscle

129. The palmar aponeurosis
1. divides into five slips distally
2. gives insertion to palmaris longus

Ans. 123. C 124. B 125. B 126. D 127. B 128. C

    3. undergoes contraction in Volkmann's ischemic contracture

    4. is related to superficial palmar arch on its deeper aspect

130. The digital synovial sheath
1. encloses only the tendon of flexor digitorum superficialis
2. extends upto the tip of the terminal phalanx
3. sheath of index finger is continuous with the ulnar bursa
4. forms vincula longa and breva to carry blood vessels to the tendons

131. The extensor expansion
1. is mainly formed by the tendon of extensor digitorum longus
2. is formed dorsal to the proximal interphalangeal joint
3. gives insertion to lumbricals and interossei
4. divides into three parts; a median part attached to the base of the terminal phalanx and two collateral parts attached to the base of the middle phalanx

132. The flexor retinaculum
1. is attached medially to the pisiform and hook of hamate
2. forms carpal tunnel through which the median and ulnar nerves pass
3. prevents buckling of tendons
4. is related superficially to the ulnar and radial arteries

133. The lateral cord of brachial plexus
1. contains fibres from the fifth, sixth and seventh cervical nerves
2. lies lateral to the axillary artery throughout
3. gives contribution to lateral pectoral, musculocutaneous and median nerves
4. is formed from the dorsal divisions of upper and middle trunks

134. The posterior cord of brachial plexus
1. is formed from the posterior divisions of all the trunks
2. lies posterior to the first and second parts of axillary artery
3. supplies mainly the muscles on the posterior aspect of upper limb
4. supplies teres major through thoracodorsal nerve

135. The ulnar nerve
1. arises from the lateral cord

Ans.   129. C 130. D 131. A 132. B 133. A 134. B

2. passes posterior to medial epicondyle of humerus
3. supplies most of the muscles of front of forearm
4. supplies all the interossei muscles

136. The median nerve
1. supplies cutaneous branches to lateral three and a half digits
2. supplies all short muscles acting on thumb
3. injury leads to ape-hand deformity
4. injury results in loss of adduction and abduction of extended fingers

137. The median nerve
1. arises from the posterior and lateral cords of brachial plexus
2. supplies muscles of front of arm
3. lies just medial to the tendon of flexor digitorum superficialis
4. passes through the carpal tunnel

138. The ulnar nerve
1. lies medial to the upper part of brachial artery
2. is accompanied by inferior ulnar collateral artery in the back of arm
3. enters the forearm between the two heads of flexor carpi ulnaris
4. supplies shoulder joint

139. The radial nerve
1. is the largest branch of the posterior cord of brachial plexus
2. gives no branch in the axilla
3. runs in the radial groove between lateral and medial heads of triceps
4. injury results in Klumpke's paralysis

140. The radial nerve supplies
1. triceps
2. anconeus
3. brachialis
4. skin over lower half of deltoid muscle

141. The ulnar nerve supplies
1. flexor carpi ulnaris
2. extensor carpi ulnaris
3. first dorsal interosseous
4. first lumbrical

Ans. 135. C 136. B 137. D 138. B 139. B 140. A 141. B

142. **The anterior interosseous nerve supplies**
   1. flexor digitorum superficialis
   2. flexor digitorum profundus
   3. pronator teres
   4. flexor pollicis longus

143. **The musculocutaneous nerve**
   1. is a branch of the lateral cord of brachial plexus
   2. passes between the two heads of biceps brachii
   3. supplies all muscles of anterior compartment of arm
   4. continues as medial cutaneous nerve of forearm

144. **The axillary artery**
   1. continues as brachial artery at the lower border of pectoralis major
   2. lies medial to the axillary vein
   3. gives lateral thoracic artery as its first branch
   4. is related throughout to brachial plexus and its branches

145. **The brachial artery**
   1. is the continuation of axillary artery at the upper border of teres major
   2. is crossed by median nerve in the middle of arm
   3. can be felt pulsating just lateral to the tendon of biceps brachii
   4. is used for measuring blood pressure

146. **The radial artery**
   1. is used for feeling pulse
   2. enters the palm between the two heads of first dorsal interosseous muscle
   3. gives princeps pollicis in the palm
   4. is the main artery forming deep palmar arch

147. **The posterior interosseous artery usually**
   1. enters the posterior compartment of forearm in company with the posterior interosseous nerve
   2. passes under the extensor retinaculum along with the extensor digitorum muscle
   3. is a branch of radial artery
   4. gives interosseous recurrent artery which anastomosis with middle collateral branch of profunda brachii artery

Ans.   142. C 143. B 144. D 145. C 146. E 147. D

148. **The basilic vein**
    1. arises from veins on the palmar aspect of hand
    2. pours most of its blood into cephalic vein through median cubital vein
    3. terminates by joining venae commitantes of brachial artery in the middle of arm
    4. continues as axillary vein at the lower border of teres major

149. **Which of the following statements are true for lymphatic drainage of the breast?**
    1. The axillary lymph nodes receive 75 percent of the lymph from the breast
    2. The parasternal lymph nodes receive lymph from both the medial and lateral halves of the breast
    3. Cancer cells from one breast can travel to the other breast through lymphatics
    4. Some lymphatics draining the upper part of mammary gland parenchyma directly go to the inferior deep cervical lymph nodes

---

Directions: Each question consists of an assertion and a reason. Responses should be choosen as follows:
    A. if the assertion and reason are true statements and the reason is a correct explanation of the assertion;
    B. if the assertion and reason are true statements but the reason is not a correct explanation of the assertion;
    C. if the assertion is true but the reason is a false statement;
    D. if the assertion is false but the reason is a true statement;
    E. if both assertion and reason are false statements.

---

150. **Fracture of the middle of the shaft of humerus results in a complete paralysis of triceps muscle**
    Because
    the radial nerve gets injured

151. **The dislocation of shoulder joint occurs primarily in the anterior direction**
    Because
    the anterior part of capsule has an opening through which the joint cavity communicates with the subscapular bursa

---

Ans.   148. D 149. E 150. D 151. D

152. **The commonest site for fracture of clavicle is at the junction of its lateral 2/3 and medial 1/3**
Because
a strong coracoclavicular ligament is attached to the lateral 1/3 of the clavicle

153. **Injury to the upper trunk of brachial plexus results in impairment of abduction at shoulder joint**
Because
it results in paralysis of deltoid and supraspinatus muscles

154. **Injury to the long thoracic nerve results in winging of scapula**
Because
scapula is retracted by the rhomboideus major and minor muscles

155. **Intramuscular injection in deltoid muscle should be given into its lower half**
Because
upper half of the muscle protects the shoulder joint

156. **When the forearm is extended and the hand supinated, its long axis is directed somewhat laterally making an angle of about 165° with the long axis of arm**
Because
the medial epicondyle of humerus is larger than the lateral epicondyle

157. **Dislocation of the elbow joint is frequently associated with fracture of upper end of ulna**
Because
whole of the olecranon process of ulna is intracapsular

158. **In small children, subluxation of the head of radius is a common occurrence**
Because
the head of radius is very small at this stage

159. **On the wrist joint, the range of abduction is more as compared to the range of adduction**
Because
there are more number of abductors than adductors acting on the wrist joint

Ans.   152. D 153. A 154. B 155. B 156. B 157. C 158. A 159. D

160. **Fracture of scaphoid is often followed by avascular necrosis of its proximal fragment**
Because
radial artery is always injured simultaneously

161. **Lunate is the commonest carpal bone to get dislocated**
Because
it takes part in the formation of the wrist joint as well as the midcarpal joint

162. **Injury to the ulnar nerve in the arm does not result in claw hand**
Because
the interossei and lumbricals are supplied by deep branch of ulnar nerve which arises in the palm

163. **Injury to the superficial branch of radial nerve affects power to supinate**
Because
the supinator and brachioradialis are paralysed

164. **Dislocation of lunate can result in loss of adduction of thumb**
Because
median nerve is pressed against the flexor retinaculum

165. **Bleeding from the deep palmar arch can be stopped by ligating ulnar artery**
Because
the deep palmar arch is mainly formed by the ulnar artery

166. **An infection of the synovial sheath within the fifth digit can spread into the fourth digit**
Because
the fourth and the fifth digits lie close to each other

167. **Injury to the recurrent branch of median nerve may result in loss of opposition of thumb**
Because
the palmar aspects of thumb and index finger will be anaesthetised

---

Ans.   160.C   161.B   162.D   163.E   164.D   165.E   166.D   167.C

168. **Axillary lymph nodes may get involved in cancer of the axillary tail of mammary gland by direct spread**
Because
the axillary tail is deep to the deep fascia and lies in close proximity to the axillary lymph nodes

169. **Basilic vein is more often used for cardiac catheterisation than the cephalic vein**
Because
most of the blood from cephalic vein is usually carried to basilic vein by the median cubital vein

170. **The median cubital vein is commonly used for blood sampling and intravenous injections**
Because
it is superficial and relatively fixed due to its communication with deep veins

171. **Injury to ulnar nerve in arm does *not* result in any cutaneous sensory loss**
Because
it does not give any branch in the arm

172. **Thecal whitlows of little finger may spread to above the wrist**
Because
the digital synovial sheath for the little finger communicates with the ulnar bursa

173. **In the case of the fracture of radius below the insertion of pronator teres the proximal fragment is pronated**
Because
the action of pronator teres is stronger than the supination action of the biceps brachii

174. **In amputation of the arm, the brachialis muscle is likely to retract more than the biceps brachii**
Because
biceps has two heads while brachialis has only one

175. **Injury to the distal epiphysial line of the humerus in a growing child will give rise to a considerable degree of shortening**

Ans.   168. A 169. D 170. A 171. D 172. A 173. E 174. B

Because
the lower end of the humerus is the growing end

176. **The swelling of hand due to edema or extravasation of blood is apparent on the dorsal aspect rather than the palmar aspect**
Because
the subcutaneous tissue is lax on the dorsal aspect

177. **Ligation of brachial artery below the origin of profunda brachii may not impair circulation through forearm**
Because
there is a rich anastomosis around elbow joint

178. **Injury to the median nerve in the middle of forearm will lead to complete loss of flexion of wrist**
Because
most of the muscles of front of forearm are supplied by the median nerve

179. **In a case of injury to the deep branch of ulnar nerve the patient will not be able to hold paper tightly between his fingers**
Because
the dorsal interossei will be paralysed

180. **An inflammatory swelling of the tendon sheath may lead to necrosis of the tendons**
Because
the swelling is likely to compress the vincular blood vessels which supply the tendons.

Ans. 175. E 176. A 177. A 178. D 179. B 180. A

CHAPTER 3

The Lower Limb

Directions: Each of the incomplete statements or questions below is followed by four or five suggested completions or answers. Select the one which is BEST in each case.

1. **The acetabulum**
   A. is directed backwards, downward and laterally
   B. is completely articular
   C. is formed by ilium and pubis only
   D. is deepened by labrum acetabulare
   E. shows a discontinuity in the superior rim, the acetabular notch

2. **The ishchiopubic rami fuse around the age of**
   A. 1 year   B. 7 year
   C. 14 year   D. 21 year

3. **Which of the following structures does *not* pass through the lesser sciatic foramen?**
   A. Internal pudendal vessels
   B. Tendon of obturator externus
   C. Pudendal nerve
   D. Nerve to obturator internus

4. **Which of the following is the most important feature of the female pelvis?**
   A. Wide and deep sciatic notch
   B. Heart shaped inlet of pelvis
   C. Subpubic angle of 90° or more
   D. Triangular obturator foramen
   E. Ischiopubic ramus is everted

Ans.   1. D   2. B   3. B   4. C

5. **The neck of the femur**
   A. is completely intracapsular
   B. is completely extracapsular
   C. has medial half intracapsular and lateral half extracapsular
   D. has anterior surface intracapsular and posterior surface extracapsular
   E. is mostly intracapsular except for its posterolateral part which is extracapsular

6. **Which of the following statements is *not* true for medial condyle of femur?**
   A. It has a larger tibial articular surface than the lateral condyle
   B. The tibial articular surface is curved
   C. It bears a groove on its medial surface for the origin of popliteus
   D. It is separated from the lateral condyle posteriorly by intercondylar notch

7. **The lower epiphyseal line of femur passes**
   A. above the adductor tubercle
   B. through the adductor tubercle
   C. below the adductor tubercle
   D. through the epicondyles of femur

8. **The adductor tubercle gives attachment to**
   A. adductor longus
   B. adductor brevis
   C. adductor magnus
   D. medial head of gastrocnemius
   E. tibial collateral ligament

9. **The medial surface of tibia**
   A. is mostly subcutaneous
   B. gives origin to tibialis anterior
   C. gives insertion to semimembranosus
   D. gives origin to sartorius, gracilis and semitendinosus
   E. has none of the above properties

10. **The bone forming the heel is**
    A. lower end of tibia   B. lower end of fibula
    C. calcaneum   D. talus

Ans.   5. E   6. C   7. B   8. C   9. A   10. C

11. **Which of the following bones does *not* take part in the medial longitudinal arch?**
    A. Calcaneum
    B. Talus
    C. Cuboid
    D. Navicular
    E. Lateral cuneiform

12. **Which of the following structures lies in the sinus tarsi?**
    A. Tendon of tibialis posterior
    B. Dorsalis paedis artery
    C. Deep peroneal nerve
    D. Interosseous talocalcaneal ligament
    E. Bifurcate ligament

13. **The patella**
    A. is a sesamoid bone which articulates with the tibia
    B. has a rough posterior surface
    C. has an apex to which ligamentum patellae is attached
    D. has a tendency for medial dislocation
    E. is surrounded on all sides by the tendon of quadriceps femoris

14. **Which of the following is *not* the growing end?**
    A. Lower end of femur
    B. Upper end of tibia
    C. Lower end of fibula
    D. Proximal end of first metatarsal

15. **The bones transmitting body weight include all the following *except***
    A. femur
    B. tibia
    C. fibula
    D. talus
    E. calcaneum

16. **Which of the following muscles is attached to lesser trochanter?**
    A. Pectineus
    B. Iliopsoas
    C. Adductor longus
    D. Adductor brevis

Ans.   11. C   12. D   13. C   14. C   15. C   16. B

17. **Which of the following structures is *not* attached to linea aspera?**
    A. Gluteus maximus
    B. Adductor longus
    C. Vastus lateralis
    D. Vastus medialis

18. **All the following statements are true regarding distal end of femur *except***
    A. it is the growing end
    B. ossification centre appears just before birth
    C. presence of ossification center has medicolegal importance
    D. articulates with tibia and fibula

19. **All the following muscles are attached to anterior surface of fibula *except***
    A. tibialis anterior
    B. extensor digitorum longus
    C. extensor hallucis longus
    D. peroneus tertius

20. **Which of the following muscles is attached to head of fibula?**
    A. Lateral head of gastrocnemius
    B. Plantaris
    C. Biceps femoris
    D. Tensor fasciae latae

21. **Which of the following muscles is *not* attached to calcaneus?**
    A. Soleus
    B. Plantaris
    C. Flexor digitorum longus
    D. Flexor digitorum accessorius

22. **How much weight is transmitted to the ground by calcaneus?**
    A. 10%
    B. 25%
    C. 50%
    D. 75%

23. **Which of the following ligaments limits adduction on hip joint?**
    A. Ischiofemoral

Ans.   17. A   18. D   19. A   20. C   21. C   22. C

B. Transverse acetabular
C. Ligamentum teres
D. Labrum acetabulare

24. **Anterior dislocation of tibia on femur is prevented by**
    A. ligamentum patellae
    B. anterior cruciate ligament
    C. posterior cruciate ligament
    D. oblique popliteal ligament

25. **Rotatory movement on knee joint occurs**
    A. between femur and menisci
    B. between tibia and menisci
    C. in both upper and lower compartments
    D. at patello-femoral joint

26. **Which of the following muscles acts on knee as well as ankle joint?**
    A. Tibialis anterior
    B. Gastrocnemius
    C. Soleus
    D. Popliteus

27. **In coxa vera**
    A. the neck-shaft angle of femur is increased
    B. the neck-shaft angle of femur is decreased
    C. the neck-shaft angle is unchanged
    D. the outer angle between thigh and leg is increased

28. **In telepes-equinovarus deformity, the foot is**
    A. plantar flexed
    B. adducted
    C. inverted
    D. shows all these features
    E. shows none of these features

29. **When the foot is on the ground, the terminal phase of extension is associated with**
    A. medial rotation of femur
    B. lateral rotation of femur
    C. medial rotation of tibia
    D. lateral rotation of tibia

Ans.   23. C   24. B   25. B   26. B   27. B   28. D   29. A

30. **In the erect posture the line of gravity falls**
    A. in front of the hip joint
    B. behind the knee joint
    C. in front of the ankle joint
    D. in front of the hip, knee and ankle
    E. behind the hip, knee and ankle

31. **The attachments of the tibial collateral ligament do *not* include**
    A. medial epicondyle of femur
    B. medial condyle of tibia
    C. medial surface of the shaft of tibia
    D. medial intercondylar tubercle of tibia
    E. medial meniscus

32. **The medial meniscus is attached to the**
    A. femur by meniscofemoral ligament
    B. tendon of popliteus
    C. anterior cruciate ligament
    D. posterior cruciate ligament
    E. none of the above

33. **The suprapatellar bursa**
    A. communicates with the knee joint occasionally
    B. lies between the quadriceps femoris muscle and anterior surface of femur
    C. is often inflammed in housemaids
    D. is pulled up by articularis genu during flexion of leg on the knee joint

34. **The superior tibio-fibular joint**
    A. is a fibrous joint
    B. is a synovial joint
    C. communicates with the knee joint
    D. allows no movement at all

35. **Which of the following is intracapsular intrasynovial?**
    A. Ligamentus teres of femur
    B. Cruciate ligaments
    C. Lateral and medial menisci
    D. Interosseous talocalcanean ligament
    E. Transverse acetabular ligament

Ans.   30. C   31. D   32. E   33. B   34. B   35. C

36. **The inferior tibio-fibular joint**
    A. communicates with the ankle joint
    B. is between the lateral and medial malleoli
    C. is a fibrous joint
    D. allows no movement at all

37. **The ankle joint is most stable in**
    A. plantar flexion
    B. dorsi flexion
    C. Inversion
    D. Eversion

38. **The quadriceps femoris is**
    A. extensor of thigh
    B. extensor of leg
    C. inserted into the apex of patella
    D. the unlocking muscle on the knee joint
    E. supplied by sciatic nerve

39. **The gluteus medius muscle**
    A. is supplied by the inferior gluteal nerve
    B. is inserted on the anterior aspect of greater trochanter
    C. is extensor of the thigh
    D. raises the pelvis of opposite side while walking
    E. is completely undercover of gluteus maximus

40. **The biceps femoris muscle**
    A. arises from hip bone only
    B. is inserted on the neck of fibula
    C. is closely related to the common peroneal nerve in popliteal fossa
    D. flexes the thigh and leg
    E. is supplied only by tibial part of sciatic nerve

41. **Which of the following muscles is extensor of both the hip and knee joints?**
    A. Hamstrings
    B. Quadriceps femoris
    C. Tensor fascia latae
    D. Gluteus medius
    E. None of the above

Ans.   36. C   37. B   38. B   39. D   40. C   41. E

42. **Which of the following muscles is flexor of both the hip and knee joints?**
    A. Biceps femoris
    B. Rectus femoris
    C. Sartorius
    D. Gracilis
    E. None of the above

43. **Which of the following muscles produces only lateral rotation of thigh?**
    A. Psoas major
    B. Adductor longus
    C. Quadratus femoris
    D. Gluteus maximus

44. **The boundaries of the femoral triangle are**
    A. inguinal ligament, sartorius and pectineus
    B. inguinal ligament, psoas major and adductor longus
    C. adductor longus, sartorius and inguinal ligament
    D. iliacus, sartorius and inguinal ligament

45. **The structures in the femoral sheath are arranged from lateral to medial side as**
    A. femoral nerve, femoral artery, femoral vein
    B. femoral artery, femoral vein, femoral canal
    C. femoral vein, femoral artery, femoral canal
    D. femoral vein, femoral artery, femoral nerve

46. **Medial boundary of femoral ring is formed by**
    A. inguinal ligament
    B. lacunar ligament
    C. pectineal ligament
    D. femoral vein

47. **All the following features pertain to gracilis muscle *except***
    A. it is attached to pubic bone
    B. it is supplied by obturator nerve
    C. it is adductor of thigh
    D. it extends the knee joint

Ans.   42. C   43. C   44. C   45. B   46. B   47. D

48. **Tensor fasciae latae**
    A. arises from anterior superior iliac spine
    B. inserted into iliotibial tract
    C. supplied by inferior gluteal nerve
    D. causes flexion on knee joint

49. **Adductor magnus muscle**
    A. is supplied by obturator and femoral nerves
    B. arises from pubic bone and ischial tuberosity
    C. is inserted into lateral lip of linea aspera
    D. causes flexion and adduction of thigh

50. **Obturator externus muscle has all the following features** *except*
    A. arises from obturator membrane
    B. inserted into trochanteric fossa
    C. supplied by obturator nerve
    D. produces medial rotation of thigh

51. **All the following structures pass under the flexor retinaculum** *except*
    A. tibialis anterior
    B. flexor hallucis longus
    C. flexor digotorum longus
    D. tibial nerve

52. **Which of the following muscles does** *not* **lie in the anterior compartment of leg?**
    A. Extensor hallucis longus
    B. Extensor digitorum longus
    C. Tibialis anterior
    D. Peroneus brevis

53. **The tendon of which of the following muscles crosses the sole from lateral to medial side?**
    A. Flexor digitorum longus
    B. Peroneus longus
    C. Tibialis posterior
    D. Flexor hallucis longus

Ans.   48. B   49. B   50. D   51. A   52. D   53. B

54. **At the apex of femoral triangle the structures are arranged from anterior to posterior side as**
    A. femoral vein, femoral artery, profunda femoris artery and profunda femoris vein
    B. femoral artery, femoral vein, profunda femoris artery and profunda femoris vein
    C. femoral vein, femoral artery, profunda femoris vein and profunda femoris artery
    D. femoral artery, femoral vein, profunda femoris vein and profunda femoris artery

55. **The articularis genu is supplied by**
    A. nerve to vastus lateralis
    B. nerve to vastus medialis
    C. nerve to vastus intermedius
    D. saphenous nerve
    E. obturator nerve

56. **Which of the following structures passes through the stem of the inferior extensor retinaculum?**
    A. Tibialis anterior
    B. Extensor digitorum longus
    C. Extensor hallucis longus
    D. Deep peroneal nerve
    E. Dorsalis paedis artery

57. **The extensor hallucis brevis**
    A. takes origin from talus
    B. is inserted into the base of the distal phalanx of big toe
    C. is supplied by superficial peroneal nerve
    D. extends the interphalangeal joint of big toe
    E. has none of the above properties

58. **When the dorsal interosseous muscle between the fourth and fifth toes contracts, it results in**
    A. extension of the metatarsophalangeal joint of the fourth toe
    B. abduction of the fifth toe
    C. adduction of the fifth toe
    D. abduction of the fourth toe
    E. flexion of the interphalangeal joint of the fourth toe

---

Ans. 54. D 55. C 56. B 57. E 58. D

59. **The movement of inversion and eversion occurs on the**
    A. ankle joint
    B. ankle and tarsometatarsal joints
    C. subtalar joint
    D. subtalar and calcaneo-cuboid joints
    E. subtalar and transverse tarsal joints

60. **Which of the following evertors is inserted into medial cuneiform and first metatarsal bone?**
    A. Peroneus longus
    B. Peroneus brevis
    C. Peroneus tertius
    D. Tibialis anterior

61. **Which of the following invertors is inserted on almost all the tarsal bones *except* talus?**
    A. Tibialis anterior
    B. Tibialis posterior
    C. Flexor hallucis longus
    D. Flexor digitorum longus

62. **The main plantar flexor on the ankle joint is**
    A. tibialis posterior
    B. flexor digitorum longus
    C. gastrocnemius
    D. peroneus longus
    E. plantaris

63. **The femoral nerve (or its branches)**
    A. supplies skin on the medial side of leg and foot
    B. supplies skin on the lateral side of thigh
    C. supplies quadratus femoris
    D. arises from the L3-L5 nerves
    E. lies within the femoral sheath

64. **The obturator nerve**
    A. arises from the sacral plexus
    B. is the sole nerve supply to pectineus
    C. enters the thigh through obturator canal
    D. injury will mainly interfere with flexion on the hip joint
    E. is purely a motor nerve

Ans.   59. E   60. A   61. B   62. C   63. A   64. C

65. **Which of the following cutaneous nerves is *not* a branch of femoral nerve?**
    A. Medial cutaneous nerve of thigh
    B. Intermediate cutaneous nerve of thigh
    C. Lateral cutaneous nerve of thigh
    D. Saphenous nerve

66. **Area of skin over upper part of femoral triangle is supplied by**
    A. ilioinguinal nerve
    B. femoral branch of genitofemoral
    C. intermediate cutaneous branch of femoral
    D. obturator nerve

67. **Accessory obturator nerve**
    A. runs along lateral pelvic wall
    B. emerges from obturator foramen
    C. supplies pectineus
    D. arises from L1 and L2 nerves

68. **Inferior gluteal nerve supplies**
    A. gluteus minimus
    B. gluteus medius
    C. gluteus maximus
    D. skin over lower part of gluteal region

69. **Muscles of anterior compartment of leg are supplied by**
    A. superficial peroneal nerve
    B. deep peroneal nerve
    C. common peroneal nerve
    D. saphenous nerve

70. **Superior gluteal nerve**
    A. has root value L4, L5, S1
    B. enters gluteal region through lesser sciatic foramen
    C. runs between gluteus maximus and gluteus medius
    D. supplies all three gluteal muscles

71. **Muscles of posterior compartment of leg are supplied by**
    A. common peroneal nerve
    B. tibial nerve

Ans.   65. C   66. B   67. C   68. C   69. B   70. A

C. sural nerve

D. all the above

72. **L4 segment of spinal cord supplies skin of**
    A. antero-lateral aspect of thigh
    B. medial aspect of leg
    C. lateral part of dorsum of foot
    D. back of thigh

73. **Tibial nerve**
    A. courses vertically down the popliteal fossa
    B. is covered throughout by skin and fascia only
    C. is accompanied by peroneal artery
    D. divides into plantar nerves behind the lateral malleolus

74. **The deep peroneal nerve**
    A. arises at the level of head of the fibula
    B. enters the anterior compartment of leg by piercing the interosseous membrane
    C. is purely a motor nerve
    D. has a terminal lateral branch ending in a pseudoganglion
    E. lies along the medial border of biceps femoris in popliteal fossa

75. **Flexion on the knee joint, after injury to the tibial part of the sciatic nerve, is done by**
    A. gastrocnemius
    B. popliteus
    C. long head of biceps femoris
    D. sartorius
    E. none of the above

76. **Foot drop is due to injury to the**
    A. superficial peroneal nerve
    B. deep peroneal nerve
    C. tibial nerve
    D. medial and lateral plantar nerves
    E. tendocalcaneus

77. **The skin on the dorsum of the foot is supplied by**
    A. saphenous nerve
    B. superficial peroneal nerve

Ans.   71. B   72. B   73. A   74. D   75. D   76. B

    C. deep peroneal nerve
    D. medial and lateral plantar nerves
    E. all the above

78. **Intramuscular injection in the gluteal region should be given in**
    A. upper medial quadrant
    B. lower medial quadrant
    C. upper lateral quadrant
    D. lower lateral quadrant
    E. its centre

79. **The medial plantar nerve supplies**
    A. flexor digitorum brevis
    B. flexor digitorum accessorius
    C. second lumbrical
    D. adductor hallucis
    E. all the above

80. **The femoral artery**
    A. is the continuation of internal iliac artery
    B. lies lateral to the femoral nerve
    C. gives profunda femoris artery
    D. leaves the femoral triangle by passing behind the adductor longus muscle
    E. supplies only the lower limb

81. **The profunda femoris artery**
    A. arises from femoral artery in adductor canal
    B. is the main artery for medial and posterior compartments of thigh
    C. leaves the adductor canal through hiatus magnus
    D. gives descending genicular artery
    E. terminates by dividing into lateral and medial circumflex arteries

82. **The posterior tibial artery**
    A. begins at the upper border of popliteus muscle
    B. gives peroneal artery which pierces the interosseous membrane
    C. divides into medial and lateral plantar arteries under the flexor retinaculum

Ans. 77. E 78. C 79. A 80. C 81. B

    D. gives nutrient artery to fibula

    E. lies deep to the tibialis posterior muscle

83. The pulsations of dorsalis paedis artery can be felt

    A. over the medial malleolus

    B. over the lateral malleolus

    C. at the distal end of first intermetatarsal space

    D. on the dorsum of foot lateral to the tendon of extensor hallucis longus

84. The dorsalis paedis artery most commonly arises from

    A. peroneal artery

    B. anterior tibial artery

    C. posterior tibial artery

    D. medial plantar artery

    E. lateral plantar artery

85. The branches of anterior tibial artery do *not* include the

    A. posterior tibial recurrent

    B. anterior tibial recurrent

    C. peroneal

    D. lateral malleolar

    E. medial malleolar

86. The great saphenous vein

    A. begins on the lateral side of foot

    B. ascends behind the medial malleolus

    C. pierces the cribriform fascia just medial to pubic tubercle

    D. is connected with deep veins through perforating veins

    E. drains only the lower limb

87. The perforating veins

    A. connect the great saphenous vein with the short saphenous vein

    B. connect the superficial veins with the deep veins

    C. normally allow passage of blood in both directions

    D. normally allow passage of blood from deep to superficial veins

    E. are mainly present in the foot

88. The commonest site for venesection of the great saphenous vein is

    A. at the saphenous opening

Ans.   82. C   83. D   84. B   85. C   86. D   87. B

    B. anterior to the medial malleolus

    C. posterior to the lateral malleolus

    D. posteromedial to the knee joint

    E. roof of popliteal fossa

89. All the following are branches of femoral artery *except*
A. superficial epigastric
B. deep circumflex iliac
C. profunda femoris
D. descending genicular

90. The obturator artery is the branch of
A. femoral artery
B. external illiac artery
C. internal iliac artery
D. profunda femoris artery

91. The popliteal artery pulse is palpated easily when
A. leg and thigh are extended
B. leg is semiflexed
C. thigh is medially rotated
D. thigh is laterally rotated

92. Which of the following vessels is used for measuring blood pressure in lower limb?
A. Femoral
B. Profunda femoris
C. Popliteal
D. Posterior tibial

93. When the back of knee joint is suddenly tapped in a standing person, he tends to fall down. Which of the following muscles is responsible for this phenomenon?
A. Quardriceps femoris
B. Biceps femoris
C. Sartorius
D. Popliteus

94. Patella has inherent tendency to dislocate laterally. The natural mechanism to prevent this is
A. long axis of femur is directed downward and medially

Ans. 88. B   89. B   90. C   91. B   92. C   93. D

   B. forward projection of medial condyle of femur
   C. attachment of vastus medialis on patella extends more distally
   D. larger articular area for patella on medial condyle of femur.

95. **All the following statements regarding fracture of tibia are true *except***
   A. common site is the junction of middle and lower thirds of tibia, being the narrowest part
   B. fractures are usually open type as most of the medial surface is subcutaneous
   C. delayed union is common because of less periosteal blood supply
   D. splint-like action of intact fibula prevents proximal and distal fragments of tibia to come in opposition.

96. **Which nerve is likely to be injured in posterior dislocation of hip joint?**
   A. Superior gluteal
   B. Perforating cutaneous
   C. Pudendal
   D. Sciatic

97. **Housemaid's knee is the inflammation of**
   A. suprapatellar bursa
   B. prepatellar bursa
   C. infrapatellar bursa
   D. synovial membrane of knee joint

98. **Weaver's bottom is the inflammation of bursa between**
   A. gluteus maximus and ischial tuberosity
   B. gluteus maximus and greater trochanter
   C. gluteus maximus and vastus lateralis
   D. adductor magnus and ischial tuberosity

99. **Which muscle is termed peripheral heart because of valveless veins present in that muscle?**
   A. Gastrocnemius
   B. Soleus
   C. Gluteus maximus
   D. Gluteus medius

Ans.   94. C   95. A   96. D   97. B   98. A   99. B

100. **Inability to extend the knee may be due to injury to**
    A. tibial nerve
    B. sciatic nerve
    C. femoral nerve
    D. obturator nerve

101. **Enlarging the femoral ring medially to relieve strangulation of femoral hernia is sometimes met with serious haemorrhage due to rupture of**
    A. femoral vein
    B. femoral artery
    C. accessory obturator artery
    D. obturator artery

102. **All the following features pertain to varicose veins** *except* **that these veins are**
    A. tortuous
    B. thickened
    C. narrowed
    D. visible

103. **All the following features point to injury to tibial nerve** *except*
    A. foot is held dorsiflexed and everted
    B. inability to stand on toes
    C. loss of sensation on sole of foot
    D. loss of sensation in back of knee

104. **Complete injury of sciatic nerve results in loss of all cutaneous sensibility below the knee** *except* **along medial side of leg and foot up to ball of big toe. This is due to intact**
    A. sural nerve
    B. saphenous nerve
    C. superficial peroneal nerve
    D. obturator nerve

105. **Which of the following muscles will escape paralysis if sciatic nerve is injured at middle level of thigh?**
    A. Hamstrings
    B. Popliteus
    C. Gastrocnemius
    D. Soleus

Ans.   100. C   101. C   102. C   103. D   104. B   105. A

Directions: For each of the incomplete statements or questions below, one or more completions or answers given is correct, Select

    A. if only 1,2 and 3 are correct;

    B. if only 1 and 3 are correct;

    C. if only 2 and 4 are correct;

    D. if only 4 is correct;

    E. if all are correct.

106. The muscles attached to the greater trochanter include

    1. obturator externus

    2. gluteus minmus

    3. gluteus medius

    4. gluteus maximus

107. The head of femur

    1. is completely intracapsular

    2. forms half the sphere

    3. gives attachment to ligamentum teres of femur

    4. is pierced by numerous vascular foramina

108. The neck of fibula

    1. is easily palpable

    2. is laterally related to anterior tibial artery

    3. gives insertion to biceps femoris

    4. when fractured, is often associated with foot drop

109. The lateral longitudinal arch is maintained by

    1. peroneus longus

    2. peroneus brevis

    3. long and short plantar ligaments

    4. small muscles of little toe

110. The medial longitudinal arch

    1. is higher than the lateral arch

    2. is less resilient than the lateral arch

    3. is maintained by tibialis posterior

    4. is flattened in pes cavus

111. The transverse tarsal joints

    1. include talonavicular and calcaneocuboid joints

    2. are fibrous joints

Ans.   106. A 107. B 108. D 109. E 110. B

3. allow movements of inversion and eversion
4. allow movements of dorsi flexion and plantar flexion

112. The fibular collateral ligament of knee joint
1. is band shaped
2. splits the tendon of biceps femoris into two parts
3. is attached to the lateral meniscus
4. is taut in extension

113. Which of the following statements is/are true for the hip joint?
1. It is a very stable, ball and socket type of synovial joint
2. Its main flexor is the iliopsoas muscle
3. Extension is limited by the iliofemoral ligament
4. It dislocates mainly anteriorly

114. In relation to the knee joint
1. it is a pure hinge type of synovial joint
2. its proximal and distal articular surfaces are congruent
3. it has no communications
4. the capsule is replaced anteriorly by the patellar retinacula, the patella and the ligamentum patellae

115. In relation to the knee joint
1. The joint cavity is divided into upper and lower compartments by the menisci
2. The movement of rotation occurs in the lower compartment
3. The collateral ligaments become taut in extension and so prevent adduction and abduction
4. The anterior cruciate ligament is attached to the lateral condyle of femur

116. In relation to the ankle joint
1. it is formed by tibia, fibula, talus and calcaneus
2. it is an ellipsoid type of synovial joint
3. tibialis posterior is the main plantar flexor
4. the main dorsiflexors are tibialis anterior and extensors of the toes

117. The deltoid ligament
1. is attached to the lateral malleolus
2. forms part of the articular surface for ankle joint

Ans. 111. B 112. C 113. A 114. D 115. E 116. D

  3. is crossed superficially by tibialis anterior
  4. is so strong a ligament that sprains of the ankle joint are very rare

118. **The spring ligament**
  1. connects the dorsal aspects of the calcaneus and the navicular bones
  2. forms part of the articular surface for head of talus in talocalcaneonavicular joint
  3. supports transverse arch of foot
  4. is supported by the tendon of tibialis posterior

119. **The blood supply to the head of femur, before fusion of its epiphysis with the diaphysis, comes from**
  1. lateral and medial circumflex femoral arteries
  2. acetabular branch of obturator artery
  3. inferior gluteal artery
  4. accetabular branch of medial circumflex femoral artery

120. **The quadriceps femoris is**
  1. supplied by the femoral nerve
  2. inserted into tibial tuberosity only
  3. the main extensor on the knee joint
  4. kept contracted in erect posture

121. **The sartorius**
  1. takes origin from the anterior inferior iliac spine
  2. lateral border forms the lateral boundary of femoral triangle
  3. is inserted into the medial border of tibia
  4. flexes the thigh as well as the leg

122. **The adductor canal**
  1. lies in the middle third of the thigh
  2. is bounded anteromedially by adductor longus and adductor magnus
  3. transmits femoral vessels
  4. transmits great saphenous vein and saphenous nerve

123. **The adductor longus muscle**
  1. has a double nerve supply
  2. is a hamstring muscle

Ans. 117. D 118. C 119. C 120. B 121. D 122. B

3. is inserted mainly into adductor tubercle
4. separates femoral vessels from profunda femoris vessels

124. The gluteus maximus
1. is supplied by the inferior gluteal nerve
2. is the main extensor on the hip joint
3. is also an extensor on the knee joint
4. is partly inserted into the gluteal tuberosity

125. The tibialis anterior
1. is inserted into all the tarsal bones except talus
2. is invertor of foot
3. is supplied by the superficial peroneal nerve
4. is an important muscle for maintenance of the medial longitudinal arch

126. The popliteus muscle
1. has intracapsular origin from the medial surface of lateral condyle of femur
2. is supplied by tibial nerve
3. unlocks the knee at the end of flexion movement
4. helps in preventing injury to the lateral meniscus

127. The flexor digitorum accessorius
1. arises from the calcaneus by two heads
2. is supplied by the medial plantar nerve
3. straightens the pull of tendon of flexor digitorum longus
4. lies directly under the plantar aponeurosis

128. Trendelenberg test is positive in
1. paralysis of gluteus maximus
2. paralysis of gluteus medius
3. paralysis of psoas major
4. dislocation of the head of femur

129. The second lumbrical muscle
1. is unipennate
2. crosses the lateral side of metatarsophalangeal joint of middle toe
3. is supplied by the digital branch of medial plantar nerve
4. is supplied by the lateral plantar nerve

Ans.   123. D 124. E 125. C 126. C 127. B 128. C 129. D

130. **The interossei muscles of the foot**
    1. consist of three dorsal interossei
    2. consist of four plantar interossei
    3. are all supplied by the deep branch of the lateral plantar nerve
    4. are so arranged that two dorsal interossei are attached to the second toe

131. **The plantar aponeurosis**
    1. resembles exactly the palmar aponeurosis
    2. is attached proximally to the calcaneus
    3. is a degenerated tendon of popliteus
    4. helps in maintaining longitudinal arches

132. **The first layer of muscles in the sole includes**
    1. adductor hallucis
    2. abductor digiti minimi
    3. flexor digitorum accessorius
    4. flexor digitorum brevis

133. **The femoral sheath**
    1. is formed by fascia iliaca anteriorly
    2. extends for about 4 cm in the thigh
    3. contains superficial inguinal lymph nodes
    4. has a medial compartment which contains connective tissue and a lymph node

134. **In relation to the femoral hernia**
    1. it is more common in males
    2. the neck of the hernial sac lies medial to the pubic tubercle
    3. coverings from within outward are femoral septum, cribriform fascia and femoral sheath
    4. the femoral ring should not be enlarged laterally to relieve strangulation

135. **The femoral artery**
    1. is not covered by any muscles in the femoral triangle
    2. continues as popliteal artery
    3. pierces the adductor magnus muscle at the junction of middle and lower thirds of the thigh
    4. can be felt pulsating at the mid-inguinal point

Ans.   130. D 131. C 132. C 133. C 134. D 135. E

136. **The popliteal artery**
    1. terminates at the upper border of the popliteus muscle
    2. runs down across the anterior surface of the popliteus muscle
    3. is crossed from medial to lateral side by the popliteal vein and the common peroneal nerve
    4. gives off several branches which participate in geniculate anastomois

137. **The lateral plantar artery**
    1. is a branch of the peroneal artery
    2. enters the sole under cover of the abductor hallucis
    3. runs deep to the flexor digitorum accessorius
    4. forms plantar arch

138. **The superficial inguinal lymphnodes drain lymph from the**
    1. lower half of the anterior abdominal wall
    2. lower part of vagina and vulva
    3. lower part of the anal canal
    4. glans penis and scrotum

139. **The lateral cutaneous nerve of thigh**
    1. is a branch of sacral plexus
    2. enters the thigh deep to the inguinal ligament
    3. supplies the gluteal region
    4. is related to a condition called meralgia paraesthetica

140. **Injury to the sciatic nerve in the gluteal region would involve**
    1. hamstring muscles
    2. all the muscles of the leg
    3. all the muscles of the foot
    4. cutaneous supply along the lateral side of leg

141. **Section of the tibial nerve may result in sensory loss along the**
    1. lateral side of leg
    2. plantar surface of heel
    3. medial border of foot on the dorsal aspect
    4. entire sole

142. **The tibial nerve**
    1. runs obliquely downwards and medially across the popliteal fossa

---

Ans.   136. D 137. C 138. A 139. C 140. E 141. C

2. crosses deep to the popliteal artery
3. supplies all the muscles of the posterior compartment of leg except plantaris
4. gives branches to the knee joint

143. The common peroneal nerve
1. has a root value of L_4-S_2
2. runs downwards and laterally along the lateral border of the biceps femoris muscle
3. supplies branches to the knee joint
4. injury would not result in any sensory loss

144. The lateral plantar nerve (or its branches)
1. supplies greater part of the skin of the sole
2. supplies most of the muscles of the sole
3. supplies all the nail beds
4. is accompanied by the lateral plantar artery which lies lateral to it

145. Loss of sensation along on the lateral border of sole may indicate injury to
1. first sacral nerve
2. second sacral nerve
3. lateral plantar nerve
4. sural nerve

Directions: Each question consists of an assertion and a reason. Responses should be choosen as follows:
   A. if the assertion and reason are true statements and the reason is a correct explanation of the assertion;
   B. if the assertion and reason are true statements but the reason is not a correct explanation of the assertion;
   C. if the assertion is true but the reason is a false statement;
   D. if the assertion is false but the reason is a true statement;
   E. if both assertion and reason are false statements.

---

146. The range of flexion of thigh on the hip joint decreases if the knee joint is kept extended
Because
the hamstring muscles cannot be stretched beyond a certain limit

---

Ans.   142. D 143. B 144. C 145. B 146. A

147. **Diseases of hip joint may result in pain in the knee joint**
Because
there are some muscles which act on both the joints

148. **Fracture at the upper end of femur is always intracapsular**
Because
the head of the femur is intracapsular

149. **In congenital dislocation of hip joint, the displacement usually takes places on to the gluteal surface**
Because
there is an opening in the posterior part of the capsule of the hip joint

150. **There is a tendency for patella to dislocate medially**
Because
the anterior projection of the lateral condyle of femur is more than that of the medial condyle

151. **Penetrating injury at the level of the apex of the femoral triangle may result in paralysis of the quadriceps femoris muscle**
Because
the femoral nerve, which is very superficial, is likely to be injured.

152. **Ligation of the femoral artery above the origin of profunda femoris artery would result in ischaemia of the lower limb**
Because
femoral artery is the main artery to supply the lower limb

153. **The adductor magnus has a double nerve supply**
Because
it is a massive muscle

154. **Injury to one inferior gluteal nerve results in lurching gait**
Because
gluteus medius muscle is paralysed

155. **In the erect posture there is minimum activity in the extensor muscles of the hip joint**
Because
flexion on the hip is prevented by the strong iliofemoral ligament

Ans. 147.B 148.D 149.C 150.D 151.E 152.D 153.B 154.E 155.C

156. **The long head of biceps femoris and the semitendinosus are flexor on the knee joint**
Because
they have a common origin from the ischial tuberosity

157. **The medial meniscus is less prone to injury**
Because
it is attached to the tibial collateral ligament

158. **Rotation on the knee joint is not at all possible**
Because
Strong collateral ligaments are present on either side of the joint

159. **Injury to the common peroneal nerve is common**
Because
it winds round the neck of fibula

160. **Injury to the tibial nerve leads to foot drop**
Because
its plantar branches supply all the muscles of sole

161. **Injury to the common peroneal nerve results in loss of dorsi flexion and eversion movements**
Because
it supplies skin on the lateral aspect of leg and dorsum of the foot

162. **Ankle joint is less stable in complete dorsiflexion**
Because
the collateral ligaments are relaxed in dorsiflexion

163. **The human foot shows longitudinal and transverse arches**
Because
arched nature of the foot provides more resilience to the foot

164. **Rupture of tendo-Achilles results in a complete loss of plantar flexion**
Because
gastrocnemius and soleus are the only plantar flexors

Ans.   156. B   157. D   158. D   159. A   160. D   161. B   162. E   163. A 164. E

165. **The range of inversion and eversion is more in plantar flexion**
Because
the narrower posterior part of the trochlear surface articulates with the tibia in this position allowing slight mobility of talus

166. **The perforating veins carry blood from deep to superficial veins**
Because
contraction of calf muscles pushes the blood into these veins

167. **Venesection and cannulation of the great saphenous vein sometimes leads to tingling sensations along the medial border of foot**
Because
the saphenous nerve is accidentally include in the ligature

168. **Fracture of the neck of femur is likely to result in avascular necrosis of the head of the femur**
Because
the head of the femur is supplied only by the retinacular arteries

169. **Intramuscular injection into the inferomedial quadrant of the gluteal region may result in foot drop**
Because
it may injure the sciatic nerve

170. **Long periods of standing predisposes to varicosities of superficial veins of lower limb**
Because
venous stasis leads to dilation of veins which reduces competency of valves

---

Ans. 165. A   166. E   167. A   168. C   169. A   170. A

CHAPTER 4

Thorax

Directions: Each of the incomplete statements or questions below is followed by four or five suggested completions or answers. Select the one which is BEST in each case.

1. **The most characteristic feature of the thoracic vertebra is**
   A. the body is heart shaped
   B. the transverse process has an articular facet for the tubercle of a rib
   C. the body has costal facets
   D. the spine is oblique

2. **Which of the following is a floating rib?**
   A. eight rib   B. ninth rib
   C. tenth rib   D. eleventh rib

3. **Which of the following ribs articulates with two vertebrae?**
   A. 1st   B. 2nd
   C. 11th   D. 12th

4. **The manubriosternal joint is a**
   A. synovial joint
   B. primary cartilaginous joint
   C. symphysis
   D. syndesmosis

5. **Which of the following statements is true about the ribs?**
   A. The first rib has outer and inner surfaces
   B. The second rib is not twisted in its long axis
   C. The seventh rib is the most oblique
   D. The middle part of each rib lies at a level lower than its vertebral end but higher than its sternal end
   E. The twelfth rib has no neck but has a shallow costal groove

---

Ans.   1. C   2. D   3. B   4. C   5. B

6. **The intercostal nerve and vessels in the costal groove are arranged from above downward as**
   A. nerve, artery and vein
   B. artery, vein and nerve
   C. vein, artery and nerve
   D. vein, nerve and artery
   E. artery, nerve and vein

7. **The upper border of sternum lies at the level of**
   A. upper border of first thoracic vertebra
   B. lower border of first thoracic vertebra
   C. upper border of second thoracic vertebra
   D. lower border of second thoracic vertebra
   E. upper border of fourth thoracic vertebra

8. **All the following features occur at the level of sternal angle *except* that**
   A. the second costal cartilage joins the sternum
   B. the superior vena cava is formed
   C. the arch of aorta begins
   D. the two pleural sacs almost meet each other
   E. the trachea bifurcates

9. **Which of the following does *not* take part in the formation of thoracic outlet?**
   A. Lower six costal cartilages
   B. Tip of xiphoid process
   C. Lower border of the 12th rib
   D. Lower border of the 12th thoracic vertebra

10. **The movements on the costovertebral joints are responsible for**
    A. increase in the anterior-posterior diameter of thorax
    B. increase in he transverse diameter of thorax
    C. increase in the vertical diameter of thorax
    D. increase in the antero-posterior and transverse diameters of thorax
    E. increase in all the three diameters of thorax

Ans.   6. C   7. D   8. B   9. B   10. D

11. **Which of the following does *not* form the boundary of inlet of thorax?**
    A. Upper border of manubrium
    B. Clavicle
    C. Upper border of 1st thoracic vertebra
    D. First costal cartilage

12. **'Bucket-handle' movement of ribs involves**
    A. movement on costo-vertebral joints
    B. raising of anterior ends of ribs
    C. increase in antero-posterior diameter of thorax
    D. elevation of sternum

13. **The most common type of accessory rib seen is**
    A. cervical
    B. lumbar
    C. bifid
    D. fused

14. **Typical intercostal space is supplied by all the following arteries *except***
    A. descending thoracic aorta
    B. internal thoracic artery
    C. musculophrenic artery
    D. thyrocervical trunk

15. **Subcostal nerve**
    A. is ventral ramus of 11th thoracic nerve
    B. enters into rectus sheath
    C. supplies 11th intercostal space
    D. supplies central part of diaphragmatic pleura

16. **The main action of the intercostal muscles is to**
    A. help in inspiration
    B. help in expiration
    C. prevent bulging out and retraction of intercostal spaces during respiration
    D. protect the underlying structures

17. **Which of the following statements is true for the intercostal muscles?**
    A. They all extend throughout the intercostal space

Ans.   11. B   12. A   13. A   14. D   15. B   16. C

    B. They arise from the upper border of the rib

    C. They are inserted into the lower border of the rib

    D. They are all supplied by the intercostal nerve of that space only

    E. They are also supplied by intercostal nerves of adjoining two spaces

18. **The first posterior intercostal artery is a branch of**

    A. descending aorta

    B. ascending aorta

    C. costocervical trunk

    D. thyrocervical trunk

    E. internal thoracic artery

19. **The posterior intercostal vein from the first right intercostal space drains into**

    A. azygos vein

    B. brachiocephalic vein

    C. subclavian vein

    D. internal thoracic vein

    E. superior intercostal vein

20. **The first intercostal nerve**

    A. arises from the dorsal ramus of the first thoracic nerve

    B. is purely sensory

    C. gives intercostobrachial nerve

    D. runs between external and internal intercostal muscles

    E. carries preganglionic sympathetic fibres for head and neck

21. **The branches of typical posterior intercostal artery do *not* include**

    A. dorsal branch

    B. collateral artery

    C. pericardiophrenic artery

    D. lateral cutaneous artery

    E. branches to the parietal pleura

22. **The contents of the posterior mediastinum do *not* include**

    A. descending aorta

    B. esophagus

    C. trachea

Ans. 17. D 18. C 19. B 20. E 21. C

D. vagus nerves
E. thoracic duct

23. Which of the following statements is *not true* about the mediastinum?
A. Its lateral boundary is formed by mediastinal pleura
B. Its anterior wall is longer than the posterior
C. Middle mediastinum contains ascending aorta and pulmonary trunk
D. In the posterior mediastinum, the esophagus crosses in front of the descending aorta
E. Mediastinum will be pushed to the right if air enters the left pleural cavity

24. Which thoracic sympathetic ganglia contribute to greater splanchnic nerves?
A. 4 to 8
B. 5 to 9
C. 6 to 10
D. 7 to 11

25. Which of the following is the largest subdivision of mediastinum?
A. Superior mediastinum
B. Inferior mediastinum
C. Middle mediastinum
D. Posterior mediastinum

26. The left mediastinal pleura is in contact with esophagus
A. in the angle between aortic arch and left subclavian artery.
B. in front of root of lung
C. between root of lung and descending aorta
D. root of neck

27. All the following statements are true for pleura *except*
A. perietal pleura is sensitive to pain
B. dips into fissures of lung
C. is mucous membrane
D. encloses a potential space

Ans.   22. C   23. B   24. B   25. B   26. A   27. C

28. **Pulmonary ligament**
    A. is part of visceral pleura
    B. contains superior pulmonary vein
    C. allows root of lung to descend during inspiration
    D. is present above the hilum

29. **The cervical pleura extends into the neck approximately**
    A. 0.5 cm above the vertebral end of the first rib
    B. 1.5 cm above the vertebral end of the first rib
    C. 2.5 cm above the vertebral end of the first rib
    D. 3.5 cm above the vertebral end of the first rib
    E. none of the above

30. **The diaphragmatic pleura is supplied by the**
    A. lower intercostal nerves
    B. phrenic nerve
    C. lower intercostal nerves and phrenic nerves
    D. sympathetic nerves
    E. parasympathetic nerves

31. **The pulmonary ligament contains**
    A. principal bronchus
    B. pulmonary artery
    C. bronchial vessels
    D. inferior pulmonary vein
    E. all the above

32. **All the following features distinguish the right lung from the left lung *except* that**
    A. it is heavier
    B. it is longer
    C. it is larger in transverse diameter
    D. it has no cardiac notch
    E. it usually has two fissures

33. **In the hilum of the right lung, the pulmonary artery lies**
    A. superior to the bronchus
    B. anterior to the bronchus
    C. inferior to the bronchus
    D. posterior to the bronchus

Ans.   28. C   29. E   30. C   31. D   32. B   33. B

34. **A bronchopulmonary segment has**
    A. an independent tertiary bronchus
    B. segmental artery
    C. veins which are intersegmental
    D. all the above properties
    E. none of the above properties

35. **Which of the following is *not* true for the bronchopulmonary segments?**
    A. The middle lobe of the right lung has two segments
    B. The medial basal segment may be absent on the left side
    C. Each segment has its own pleural covering
    D. Some diseases may be localised to one segment
    E. Surgical removal of a segment is possible

36. **The mediastinal surface of the left lung is *not* directly related to the**
    A. esophagus
    B. trachea
    C. descending aorta
    D. thoracic duct
    E. right ventricle

37. **All the following nerves supply lungs *except***
    A. vagus
    B. sympathetic trunk
    C. phrenic
    D. pulmonary plexus

38. **Pericardium is supplied by all the following *except***
    A. phrenic nerve
    B. vagus
    C. cardiac plexuses
    D. 2nd-6th intercostal nerves

39. **Epicardium consists of**
    A. cardiac muscle
    B. inner lining of heart
    C. visceral pericardium
    D. fibrous pericardium

Ans.   34. D   35. C   36. B   37. C   38. D   39. C

40. **Base of the heart is mainly formed by**
   A. right atrium
   B. left atrium
   C. right ventricle
   D. left ventricle

41. **Diaphragmatic surface of heart is formed by**
   A. right ventricle and right atrium
   B. left ventricle and left atrium
   C. right atrium and left atrium
   D. left ventricle and right ventricle

42. **Which of the following does *not* form a feature of ventricles?**
   A. Trabeculae carnae
   B. Papillary muscle
   C. Musculi pectinati
   D. Chordae tendinae

43. **Great cardiac vein**
   A. begins at the base of heart
   B. lies in anterior interventricular groove
   C. joins right end of coronary sinus
   D. receives veins from right atrium

44. **Which of the following statements is *not* true for the surfaces of heart?**
   A. The sternocostal surface is mainly formed by the two ventricles
   B. The diaphragmatic surface is formed by the two ventricles and the left atrium
   C. The base is formed mainly by the left atrium
   D. The left surface is formed by the left auricle and the left ventricle

45. **The right border of the heart is formed by the**
   A. right ventricle
   B. right atrium
   C. right auricle
   D. right atrium and right ventricle
   E. right auricle and right ventricle

46. **Which of the following openings is not guarded by any valve?**
   A. Inferior vena cava

Ans.   40. B   41. D   42. C   43. B   44. B   45. B

    B. Coronary sinus
    C. Pulmonary trunk
    D. Pulmonary vein
    E. Ascending aorta

47. Which of the following does *not* open in the right atrium?
    A. Superior vena cava
    B. Inferior vena cava
    C. Mitral orifice
    D. Coronary sinus
    E. Anterior cardiac vein

48. The atrioventricular node
    A. is made up of ordinary cardiac muscle
    B. is usually supplied by the left coronary artery
    C. is a pacemaker of heart
    D. lies in the interatrial septum
    E. lies in the membranous part of the interventricular septum

49. All the following veins terminate in the coronary sinus *except* the
    A. great cardiac
    B. middle cardiac
    C. small cardiac
    D. anterior cardiac
    E. oblique vein of left atrium

50. In a plain antero-posterior radiograph the left margin of the mediastinal shadow in formed by
    A. arch of aorta
    B. pulmonary trunk
    C. left auricle
    D. left ventricle
    E. all the above

51. The descending thoracic aorta gives origin to
    A. all the posterior intercostal arteries
    B. coronary arteries
    C. esophageal arteries
    D. pericardiophrenic artery
    E. branches to thymus

Ans.   46. D   47. C   48. D   49. D   50. E   51. C

52. **All the following statements are true about the ascending aorta *except* that**
    A. it lies anterior to the transverse sinus of pericardium
    B. its opening is guarded by a valve with three semilunar cusps
    C. its opening lies to the left of the pulmonary orifice
    D. it gives coronary arteries
    E. it is covered by serous as well as fibrous pericardium

53. **All the following statements are true about the brachiocephalic trunk *except* that**
    A. it is the first branch of the arch of aorta
    B. it divides into the right and left common carotid arteries
    C. it is crossed by the left brachiocephalic vein
    D. it ascends at first in front of and then to the right of trachea
    E. it bifurcates behind the right sternoclavicular joint

54. **The internal thoracic artery is the branch of**
    A. brachiocephalic trunk
    B. first part of the subclavian artery
    C. second part of the subclavian artery
    D. axillary artery
    E. costocervical trunk

55. **Which of the following is *not* a branch of the internal thoracic artery?**
    A. Perforating artery
    B. Superior epigastric artery
    C. Musculophrenic artery
    D. Pericardiophrenic artery
    E. Superior intercostal artery

56. **Which of the following structures crosses anterior and left surface of the arch of aorta?**
    A. Left brachiocephalic vein
    B. Left recurrent laryngeal nerve
    C. Left phrenic nerve
    D. Trachea
    E. Thoracic duct

57. **All the following are the branches of the arch of aorta *except* the**
    A. left common carotid

Ans.   52. C   53. B   54. B   55. E   56. C

    B. right common carotid
    C. brachiocephalic trunk
    D. left subclavian
    E. thyroidea ima

58. All the following structures lie anterior to the descending thoracic aorta *except* the
    A. left bronchus
    B. pericardium
    C. terminal part of hemiazygos veins
    D. esophagus
    E. diaphragm

59. Which of the following is a direct tributary of the superior vena cava?
    A. Right internal jugular vein
    B. Azygos vein
    C. Hemiazygos vein
    D. Internal thoracic vein
    E. Right superior intercostal vein

60. The superior intercostal vein is usually formed by the union of posterior intercostal veins of
    A. Ist and 2nd intercostal spaces
    B. Ist to 3rd intercostal spaces
    C. 2nd to 4th intercostal spaces
    D. 3rd and 4th intercostal spaces
    E. 3rd to 5th intercostal spaces

61. The azygos vein receives all the following veins *except* the
    A. ascending lumbar vein
    B. first posterior intercostal vein
    C. hemiazygos vein
    D. right bronchial veins
    E. accessory hemiazygos vein

62. The tracheal bifurcation
    A. lies in the median plane
    B. lies to the left of the median plane
    C. moves down with inspiration
    D. lies at the level of first costal cartilage

Ans.   57. B   58. C   59. B   60. C   61. B   62. C

63. All the following structures form anterior relations of the trachea *except* the
    A. isthmus of thyroid gland
    B. inferior thyroid veins
    C. arch of aorta
    D. arch of vena azygos
    E. origin of the left common carotid artery

64. All the following structures from anterior relations of the esophagus except the
    A. trachea
    B. pericardium and left atrium
    C. right pulmonary artery
    D. descending thoracic aorta
    E. left principal bronchus

65. The gastroesophageal junction lies at the level of
    A. left nipple
    B. xiphisternal junction
    C. 8th costal cartilage
    D. upper end of linea semilunaris
    E. none of the above

66. Which of the following statements is true about the nerve supply of heart?
    A. The deep cardiac plexus is formed by superior cervical cardiac branch of left sympathetic trunk and inferior cervical cardiac branch of left vagus
    B. The superficial cardiac plexus lies in front of the bifurcation of trachea
    C. The sympathetic fibres slow the rate of discharge from the sinoatrial node
    D. The sympathetic fibres dilate the coronary arteries
    E. The parasymapathetic fibres carry pain sensations from heart

67. The thoracic duct
    A. has no valves
    B. ascends behind the esophagus in the posterior mediastinum
    C. lies to the left of trachea in the superior mediastinum

---

Ans. 63. D 64. D 65. E 66. D

D. drains the lymph from the entire body except the right upper limb and the right half of head and neck

68. **All the following statements are true about aortic sinuses** *except*
A. these are three dilatations
B. are located opposite the aortic cusps
C. give origin to right and left interventricular arteries
D. are found at the origin of the ascending aorta

69. **All the following statements are true for thymus** *except*
A. is necessary for development of lymphoid tissue in newborn
B. produces immunologically competent lymphocytes
C. lies in posterior mediastinum
D. involutes after puberty

70. **Which of the following statements regarding collateral circulation after superior vena cava obstruction is** *not* **correct?**
A. Azygos vein forms the collateral route
B. Vertebral venous plexus forms the collateral route
C. Caput medusae forms the collateral route
D. Thoracoepigastric vein forms the collateral route

71. **After abdominal operations, infants are susceptible to lung infection (pneumonia). All the following anatomical factors play a role** *except*
A. ribs are horizontal so pump handle movement is not possible
B. respiration in infants is purely abdominal
C. post-operative pain restricts respiration and secretions accumulate in lungs
D. cough reflex is not developed in infants to cough out the secretions from lungs

72. **All the following statements regarding 'Paracentasis thoracis' (aspiration from pleural cavity) are true** *except*
A. thoracic wall upto parietal pleura is to be anaesthetised
B. aspiration needle is inserted in lower part of intercostal space
C. needle is inserted in mid-axillary line
D. costo-diaphragmatic recess is narrowed in mid-axillary line

73. **The site chosen for 'pericardiocentesis' (aspiration from pericardial cavity) is**
A. left 3rd intercostal space

Ans.   67. B   68. C   69. C   70. C   71. D   72. D

      B. right 4th intercostal space

      C. left 5th intercostal space

      D. right costo-xiphoid angle

74. **Penetrating injury just below the costal margin at all the following sites may injure pleura** *except*

      A. right costo-vertebral angle

      B. left costo-vertebral angle

      C. right costo-xiphoid angle

      D. left costo-xiphoid angle

75. **The vessel usually chosen for coronary by-pass operation to overcome obliteration of coronary artery is**

      A. great saphenous vein

      B. cephalic vein

      C. left gastroepiphoic artery

      D. internal thoracic artery

76. **All the following statements regarding coronary circulation are true** *except*

      A. coronary arteries are anatomical end-arteries.

      B. gradual obliteration of coronaries allows development of collaterals

      C. exercise increases collateral circulation

      D. collateral channels develop with ageing.

77. **Which of the following statements regarding phrenic nerve is correct?**

      A. It arises from brachial plexus

      B. It enters the thorax by crossing behind the subclavian artery

      C. It runs anterior to the root of lung

      D. If injured the dome of diaphragm falls to a lower level on that side.

78. **Which of the following statements concerning blood supply to heart is** *not* **correct?**

      A. Coronary arteries are branches of ascending aorta

      B. Circumflex artery runs in the anterior inter-ventricular groove

      C. S.A. node is usually supplied by right coronary artery

      D. Occlusion of a coronary artery can result in arrhythmias.

Ans.   73. C   74. D   75. D   76. A   77. C   78. B

79. In a person the ventricles start beating independently of the atria at a slower rate. This could be due to occlusion of
   A. posterior interventricular artery
   B. anterior interventricular artery
   C. marginal artery
   D. conus artery

80. If a rib is fractured at two nearby places, the part of rib between two fractured sites will show which of the following features?
   A. Move outward during inspiration
   B. Move inward during inspiration
   C. Move inward during expiration
   D. Does not move at all

81. All the following statements regarding bronchopulmonary segments are true *except*
   A. each is supplied by a tertiary bronchiole
   B. they are separated by intersegmental veins
   C. they are drained by pulmonary lymphnodes
   D. many diseases are localised to a particular segment

Directions: For each of the incomplete statements or questions below, one or more completions or answers given is correct. Response should be choosen as follows:
   A. if one 1,2 and 3 are correct;
   B. if only 1 and 3 are correct;
   C. if only 2 and 4 are correct;
   D. if only 4 is correct;
   E. if all are correct.

---

82. The features of the twelfth thoracic vertebra include
   1. one complete costal facet and one demifacet on the side of the body
   2. presence of mamillary processes
   3. long transverse processes
   4. inferior articular facets facing forward and laterally

83. The features of the twelfth rib include
   1. broad anterior end bearing a tapering costal cartilage
   2. no costal groove

Ans. 79. A   80. B   81. A   82. D

3. tubercle having articular and non-articular parts
4. inner surface facing inwards and upwards

84. The 12th rib
1. gives insertion to the quadratus lumborum muscle
2. gives origin to the diaphragm
3. is related to pleura in its medial half
4. gives attachment to the medial arcuate ligament

85. The manubrium sterni
1. articulates with the clavicle and the first two costal cartilages only
2. is not related to pleura
3. is directly related to trachea on its posterior aspect
4. is used for taking bone marrow samples

86. The first rib
1. articulates posteriorly with the first thoracic vertebra only
2. is united to the clavicle by a ligament
3. is not easily palpable
4. shows two grooves on its upper surface; the posterior groove is related to the subclavian vein and the lower trunk of brachial plexus

87. The internal intercostal muscle
1. extends from the angle of the rib to the sternum
2. is related to the intercostal nerve and vessels on its superficial aspect
3. is replaced posteriorly by the posterior intercostal membrane
4. is pierced by branches which supply parietal pleura

88. The right pleura
1. lies in the median plane from jugular notch to the xiphisternal joint
2. extends upto the sixth rib in the mid-clavicular line
3. does not extend below the level of the 12th rib
4. is separated from the left pleura posteriorly by a distance approximately equal to the width of the bodies of thoracic vertebrae

89. The visceral pleura
1. lines the fissures separating various lobes

Ans. 83. C   84. A   85. D   86. A   87. B   88. D

2. separates bronchopulmonary segments from each other
3. is relatively insensitive to pain
4. covering the apex of lung is called cervical pleura

90. In abdominal incisions pleura is likely to be injured in
1. right costovertebral angle
2. left costovertebral angle
3. right xiphicostal angle
4. left xiphicostal angle

91. Cancer of left lung may involve
1. right tracheobronchial lymph nodes
2. left tracheobronchial lymph nodes
3. left hilar lymph nodes
4. left axillary lymph nodes

92. The mediastinal surface of the right lung
1. is related to the right atrium posterio-inferior to the hilus
2. is separated from the trachea by the right vagus and the arch of vena azygos
3. shows both segments of the middle lobe
4. is related to the ascending aorta

93. In relation to the blood supply of lungs the
1. right bronchial arteries arise directly from the descending thoracic aorta
2. left bronchial arteries arise from the descending thoracic aorta
3. right bronchial veins open into right superior intercostal vein
4. left bronchial veins open into left superior intercostal vein

94. The fibrous pericardium
1. has visceral and parietal layers
2. is fused with the central tendon of diaphragm
3. contains heart, ascending aorta, arch of aorta and superior vena cava
4. is supplied by the phrenic nerves

95. In relation to the serous pericardium
1. the oblique sinus lies behind the left atrium
2. the ascending aorta and pulmonary trunk are enclosed in separate sleeves of serous pericardium

---

Ans.   89. B   90. A   91. A   92. C   93. C   94. C

3. the oblique sinus opens inferiorly and to the left
4. is insensitive to pain

96. The left atrium
1. mainly forms the left border of heart
2. has smooth walls except in the auricle
3. lies anterior to the transverse sinus of pericardium
4. has openings of four pulmonary veins

97. In relation to the left ventricle
1. the cavity is circular in cross section
2. there are two main papillary muscles
3. the walls are three times thicker than those of the right ventricle
4. the entire ventricle is rough due to the presence of trabeculae carnae

98. The left ventricle
1. forms the sternocostal surface and the base of the heart
2. is supplied by left coronary artery only
3. has a moderator band
4. pumps blood equal in volume to that pumped by the right ventricle

99. In relation to the mitral valve
1. it has two cusps
2. the anterior cusp is larger than the posterior cusp
3. both the cusps are attached to both the papillary muscles by chordae tendinae
4. blood flows on both surfaces of the posterior cusp

100. The aortic opening
1. lies anterior and to the left of the pulmonary opening
2. is guarded by a valve having one anterior and two posterior cusps
3. lies at the level of the 3rd costal cartilage
4. lies at the level of the 3rd intercostal space

101. In relation to the right ventricle the
1. infundibulum is the upper smooth part of the ventricle
2. papillary muscles are three in number

Ans. 95. B 96. C 97. A 98. D 99. A 100. C

3. anterior papillary muscle sends chordae tendinae to the anterior and the posterior cusps
4. moderator band carries bundle of His

102. The interatrial septum
1. lies in the median plane
2. shows fossa ovalis on its right surface
3. shows musculi pectinati
4. contains atrioventricular node

103. The interventricular septum
1. is made up of muscular and membranous parts
2. presents no trabeculae carnae
3. separates the right atrium and right ventricle from the left ventricle
4. bulges towards the left ventricle

104. The apex beat
1. is usually felt in the 5th left intercostal space
2. lies medial to the midclavicular line
3. is often visible
4. indicates the position of the apex of heart

105. The sinuatrial node
1. is present at the lower end of the crista terminalis
2. is connected to the atrioventricular node by the purkinje fibres
3. gives origin to the atrioventricular bundle
4. is usually supplied by the right coronary artery

106. The bundle of His
1. is also called the moderator band
2. divides at the upper margin of the membranous part of interventricular septum
3. lies within the interatrial septum
4. lies within the interventricular septum

107. The right coronary artery
1. arises from the anterior aortic sinus
2. gives anterior interventricular branch
3. runs in the right part of coronary sulcus
4. supplies most of the inteventricular septum

Ans.   101. A 102. C 103. B 104. E 105. D 106. D 107. B

108. **The left coronary artery**
  1. arises from the anterior aortic sinus
  2. lies between the pulmonary trunk and the left atrium
  3. gives posterior interventricular branch
  4. supplies part of the right ventricle also

109. **The anterior interventricular artery**
  1. is the branch of the left coronary artery
  2. runs in the coronary sulcus
  3. winds round the inferior border of heart to enter the posterior interventricular groove
  4. is accompanied by the middle cardiac vein

110. **The coronary sinus**
  1. drains the entire blood from the heart
  2. lies in the posterior and left part of the coronary sulcus
  3. is accompanied by the left coronary artery
  4. opens into the right atrium

111. **The opening of the coronary sinus**
  1. lies in the left atrium
  2. lies between the inferior vena caval and the right atriventricular openings
  3. lies in the rough part of the right atrium
  4. is guarded by a valve

112. **The pulmonary trunk**
  1. arises from the infundibulum of right atrium
  2. bifurcates into pulmonary veins
  3. lies within the fibrous pericardium but outside the serous pericardium
  4. lies anterior and to the left of the beginning of the ascending aorta

113. **The arch of aorta**
  1. begins behind the right half of the sternal angle
  2. lies almost in coronal plane
  3. grooves the esophagus
  4. reaches upto the jugular notch

Ans.   108. C   109. B   110. C   111. C   112. D   113. B

114. **Which of the following statements are true for the relations of the arch of aorta?**
1. Its posterior and right surface is related to the trachea and esophagus
2. Its anterior and left surface is related to the left lung and pleura
3. It is related superiorly to the left brachiocephalic vein
4. It is related inferiorly to the ligamentum arteriosum

115. **The descending thoracic aorta**
1. in its upper part lies to the left of the vertebral column
2. lies at first to the left of and then behind the esophagus
3. pierces the diaphragm in the median plane
4. bulges into the left pleural cavity producing a distinct groove on the left lung

116. **The internal thoracic artery**
1. lies under cover of the margin of sternum
2. terminates in the third intercostal space
3. is throughout accompanied by the internal thoracic vein
4. supplies mammary gland

117. **The superior vena cava**
1. is formed at the level of 2nd costal cartilage
2. grooves the right lung
3. pierces the pearicardium just before opening into the right atrium
4. receives azygos vein at the level of sternal angle

118. **The superior vena cava**
1. is formed by the union of right and left brachiocephalic veins
2. lies lateral to the right phrenic nerve
3. forms posterior boundary of the transverse sinus of pericardium
4. lies undercover of the sternum

119. **The azygos vein**
1. begins at the level of second lumbar vertebra
2. enters the thorax through the aortic opening
3. connects superior and inferior venae cavae
4. has brachiocephalic veins as its principal tributaries

Ans.   114. E   115. E   116. D   117. C   118. B   119. A

120. **The inferior hemiazygos vein**
    1. arises from the left renal vein
    2. begins by the union of the left ascending lumbar vein and the left subcostal vein
    3. receives lower three or four left posterior intercostal veins
    4. passes anterior to the descending aorta to terminate in the azygos vein

121. **The direct tributaries of left brachiocephalic vein are**
    1. thoracic duct
    2. left inferior thyroid vein
    3. left superior intercostal vein
    4. left bronchial veins

122. **The trachea**
    1. is in the median plane at the inlet of thorax
    2. is deviated to the right at its termination
    3. is lying anterior to the esophagus
    4. lies in the superior and posterior mediastinum

123. **The cervical part of trachea**
    1. is related on either side to the carotid sheath
    2. is related on either side to the thyroid gland
    3. is related anteriorly to the isthmus of thyroid gland
    4. has a cartilage called carina at its upper end

124. **The right principal bronchus differs from the left principal bronchus in being**
    1. wider
    2. more oblique
    3. shorter
    4. less prone to receive foreign bodies

125. **The esophagus**
    1. begins at the upper border of cricoid cartilage
    2. runs a straight course throughout
    3. is narrowest at its termination
    4. is narrowest at its begining

126. **The esophagus**
    1. has a small collapsed lumen except during deglutition

Ans.   120. A 121. A 122. A 123. A 124. B 125. D

 2. remains is contact with the vertebral column throughout its course
 3. is supplied by inferior thyroid vessels, direct branches of aorta and left gastric vessels
 4. shows three constrictions

127. The esophagus
 1. has a functional sphincter mechanism at its lower end
 2. measures about 25 cm
 3. pierces through the right crus of diaphragm
 4. enters the stomach at the level of xiphisternal joint

128. The esophagus
 1. has smooth muscle only
 2. is separated from the mediastinal surface of the left lung by the arch of aorta
 3. is drained by systemic veins only
 4. is crossed posteriorly by the thoracic duct

129. The thoracic duct
 1. is about 40 cm long
 2. begins from cisterna chyli
 3. enters the thorax through the aortic orifice of the diaphragm
 4. ascends upto the level of the transverse process of the seventh cervical vertebra before terminating into the left brachiocephalic vein

130. The superficial cardiac plexus
 1. lies infront of the ligamentum arteriosum
 2. is formed by the inferior cervical cardiac branch of the left sympathetic trunk
 3. is formed by the inferior cervical cardiac branch of the left vagus
 4. receives contribution from the recurrent laryngeal nerves

131. In relation to the thoracic part of the sympathetic trunk
 1. there are twelve ganglia
 2. all the ganglia contribute branches to the aortic plexus
 3. each ganglion is connected to the ventral ramus of the corresponding thoracic nerve by a grey and a white ramus communicans

Ans.   126. B   127. A   128. C   129. E   130. B

4. the white ramus joins the nerve proximal to the attachment of the gray ramus communicans

132. **The lesser splanchnic nerve**
    1. is formed by the branches of 9th and 10th thoracic sympathetic ganglia
    2. lies lateral to the sympathetic trunk
    3. pierces through the crus of the diaphragm
    4. mainly consists of postganglionic fibres

Directions: Each question consists of an assertion and a reason. Responses should be choosen as follows:
    A. if the assertion and reason are true statements and the reason is a correct explanation of the assertion;
    B. if the assertion and reason are true statements but the reason is not a correct explanation of the assertion;
    C. if the assertion is true but the reason is a false statement;
    D. if the assertion is false but the reason is a true statement;
    E. if both assertion and reason are false statements.

---

133. **The first rib and the manubrium sterni move as a unit during respiration**
    Because
    these two bones are connected by an immovable fibrous joint

134. **The bucket handle movement of ribs results in an increase in the antero-posterior diameter of the thorax**
    Because
    the sternal end of the rib lies at a lower level than its vertebral end

135. **The left border of the heart can be marked out by light percussion**
    Because
    it is not covered by the lung due to the presence of cardiac notch

136. **Blockage of a branch of coronary artery leads to myocardial necrosis in the area supplied by that branch**
    Because
    the anastomosis between coronary arteries are insufficient

---

Ans. 131. B 132. B 133. C 134. D 135. E 136. A

137. **The inteventricular septum bulges towards the right ventricle**
Because
more blood enters the left ventricle as compared to the right ventricle

138. **Inflammation of the peripheral part of diaphragmatic pleura may result in pain in the shoulder region**
Because
the diaphragm and the skin over shoulder region are supplied by the same segments of the spinal cord

139. **A puncture in the intercostal space should be made near the lower border of the rib**
Because
the lower border of the rib is thinner than the upper border

140. **In case of pleural effusion, the fluid first accumulates in the costodiaphragmatic recess**
Because
this is the most dependent part of the pleural cavity when the person is ambulatory

141. **Stab wounds immediately above the medial third of the clavicle cannot injure the pleura**
Because
the cervical pleura is protected by suprapleural membrane

142. **The cartilages in the trachea are absent posteriorly**
Because
posteriorly muscle fibres are present which can change the diameter of trachea

143. **Foreign bodies from trachea tend to go the left bronchus**
Because
the left bronchus is wider and more in line with the trachea

144. **The walls of the right ventricle are thicker than those of the left ventricle**
Because
the right artrioventricular orifice is larger than the left atrioventricular orifice

---

Ans.   137. C 138. D 139. D 140. A 141. B 142. B 143. E 144.D

145. Each thoracic sympathetic ganglion is connected to the intercostal nerve by both the white and the gray rami communicans
Because
the preganglionic sympathetic neurons are present in all the thoracic segments of the spinal cord

146. **In a plain posterio-anterior skiagram of chest, enlargement of left atrium cannot be appreciated**
Because
the left atrium hardly forms the sternocostal surface of heart

---

Ans. 145. A **146. A**

CHAPTER 5

Abdomen

Directions: Each of the incomplete statements or questions below is followed by four or five suggested completions or answers. Select the one which is BEST in each case.

1. **Which of the following does *not* form a surface landmark?**
    A. Pubic tubercle
    B. Pecten pubis
    C. Anterior superior iliac spine
    D. Tubercle of iliac crest
    E. Iliac crest

2. **Structures attached to the pubic tubercle do *not* include the**
    A. inguinal ligament   B. lacunar ligament
    C. linea alba   D. reflected inguinal ligament
    E. cremaster muscle

3. **The ilium, ischium and pubis fuse with each other at the age of**
    A. one year   B. eight year
    C. puberty   D. 15-25 years
    E. 40 years

4. **The highest point of the iliac crest lies at the level of the interval between spines of the**
    A. first and second lumbar vertebrae
    B. second and third lumbar vertebrae
    C. third and fourth lumbar vertebrae
    D. fourth and fifth lumbar vertebrae
    E. fifth lumbar and first sacral vertebrae

Ans.   1. B   2. C   3. D   4. C

5. **Which of the joints of pelvis is synovial type?**
   A. Pubic symphysis
   B. Sacroiliac
   C. Lumbosacral
   D. Sacrococcygeal

6. **In the anatomical position of pelvis**
   A. pelvic surface of body of pubis faces backwards.
   B. pelvic surface of sacrum faces forwards.
   C. plane of pelvic inlet makes an angle of 15°-20° with horizontal.
   D. anterior superior iliac spine and pubic tubercle lie in the same coronal plane.

7. **Lymphatic drainage of lower half of anterior abdominal wall is into**
   A. lumbar nodes
   B. aortic nodes
   C. axillary nodes
   D. inguinal nodes

8. **All the following statements regarding fascia transversalis are false** *except*
   A. forms the posterior wall of rectus sheath
   B. prolonged as posterior wall of femoral sheath
   C. prolonged as external spermatic fascia
   D. lies deep to transversus abdominis

9. **Conjoint tendon**
   A. formed by fusion of aponeurosis of internal and external oblique muscles.
   B. continues medially with the posterior wall of rectus sheath.
   C. attached to iliopubic eminence.
   D. strengthens medial part of posterior wall of inguinal canal.

10. **Medial arcuate ligament bridges over**
    A. right crus of diaphragm
    B. quadratus lumborum
    C. psoas major
    D. pectineus

Ans. 5. B   6. D   7. D   8. D   9. D   10. C

11. **The internal oblique muscle of abdomen**
    A. takes origin from the lower six costal cartilages
    B. forms posterior rectus sheath only
    C. has tripple relation with the inguinal canal
    D. extends as internal spermatic fascia on the spermatic cord
    E. is not supplied by the first lumbar nerve

12. **A little above the pubis, the posterior rectus sheath is formed by**
    A. aponeurosis of internal oblique
    B. aponeurosis of transversus abdominis
    C. fascia transversalis
    D. peritoneum
    E. none of the above

13. **The contents of the rectus sheath do *not* include the**
    A. pyramidalis muscle
    B. superior epigastric vessels
    C. inferior epigastric vessels
    D. iliohypogastric nerve
    E. subcostal nerve

14. **The rectus abdominis muscle**
    A. arises from the pubic crest and the pubic tubercle
    B. usually shows five tendinous intersections
    C. is supplied by the lower six thoracic and the first lumbar nerves
    D. is adherent to the posterior rectus sheath in the region of tendinous intersections
    E. flexes the vertebral column

15. **All the following structures pass through the deep inguinal ring *except* the**
    A. ductus deferens
    B. testicular artery
    C. pampiniform plexus of veins
    D. ilioinguinal nerve
    E. genital branch of genito femoral nerve

16. **The posterior wall of the inguinal canal is formed by all the following structures *except* the**
    A. fascia transversalis

Ans.   11. C   12. E   13. D   14. E   15. D

B. conjoint tendon
C. lacunar ligament
D. reflected part of inguinal ligament

17. **The spinal nerve supplying the skin around the umbilicus is the**
    A. ninth thoracic
    B. tenth thoracic
    C. twelfth thoracic
    D. first lumbar
    E. third lumbar

18. **The neurovascular plane in the anterior abdominal wall is between**
    A. the external oblique and the internal oblique
    B. the external oblique and the transversus abdominis
    C. the internal oblique and the transversus abdominis
    D. the transversus abdominis and the fascia transversalis
    E. the fascia transversalis and the parietal peritoneum

19. **Which of the following statements is not true about the actions of muscles of the anterior abdominal wall?**
    A. They contract in inspiration
    B. They help in expiration
    C. They help in increasing intrabdominal pressure
    D. They help in flexing and rotating the vertebral column
    E. They oppose the action of gravity on abdominal viscera in erect posture

20. **The quadratus lumborum muscle**
    A. arises from the dorsal segment of iliac crest
    B. is enclosed between the posterior and the middle layers of the thoracolumbar fascia
    C. fixes the 12th rib in inspiration
    D. flexes the vertebral column forwards
    E. is supplied by the dorsal rami of lumbar nerves

21. **The pelvic diaphragm**
    A. is formed by the two levator ani muscles only
    B. is pierced by the uterus
    C. forms an important support for the pelvic viscera

Ans. 16. C   17. B   18. C   19. A   20. C

D. is supplied by the branches from the lumbar plexus
E. is pierced by nerves and vessels going to the perineum

22. The diaphragm
A. has a sternal origin from the posterior surface of the lower end of the body of sternum
B. has two crura attached to the lumbar vertebrae
C. has a central tendon which is pierced by the esophagus
D. is inserted into the lower six costal cartilages
E. receives its motor innervation from the phrenic and the lower intercostal nerves

23. The inferior vena caval opening in the diaphragm
A. lies at the level of the 10th thoracic vertebra
B. lies in the central tendon of diaphragm
C. does not transmit any other structure
D. also transmits the right vagus nerve
E. is uneffected by diaphragmatic contraction

24. True statement in relation to innervation of the diaphragm is that the
A. lower intercostal nerves supply sensory fibres to the whole of the diaphragm
B. phrenic nerve carries motor as well as sensory fibres
C. phrenic nerve carries only motor fibres
D. sympathetic nerves supply sensory fibres
E. spinal segments C3, C4 and C5 constitute the only source

25. The diaphragm is at the lowest level in
A. standing position
B. sitting position
C. supine position
D. prone position

26. Which of the following lies in the gastrosplenic ligament?
A. Splenic artery
B. Left gastric artery
C. Left gastroepiploic vessels
D. Tail of pancreas
E. Splenic vein

Ans.   21. C   22. B   23. B   24. B   25. B   26. C

27. Which of the following ligaments is *not* connected to the liver?
    A. Triangular ligament
    B. Coronary ligament
    C. Falciform ligament
    D. Lienorenal ligament
    E. Lesser omentum

28. Which of the following is *not* a part of the lesser sac?
    A. Superior recess
    B. Splenic recess
    C. Inferior recess
    D. Paraduodenal recess
    E. Vestibule

29. Which of the following statements is *not* true for the mesentery of the small intestine?
    A. Its root is only about 6 inches long
    B. It extends from the left side of L2 vertebra to the right sacroiliac joint
    C. It crosses successively third part of duodenum, aorta, and inferior vena cava
    D. It contains inferior mesenteric vessels
    E. It contains about a hundred lymph nodes

30. The duodenojejunal flexure is fixed to the posterior abdominal wall by the
    A. falciform ligament
    B. ligament of Treitz
    C. hepatoduodenal ligament
    D. lesser omentum
    E. greater omentum

31. All the following ligments are attached to the greater curvature of the stomach *except* the
    A. gastrophrenic
    B. gastrosplenic
    C. gastrohepatic
    D. greater omentum

32. Visceral surface of liver is related to all the following *except*
    A. stomach

Ans.   27. D   28. D   29. D   30. B   31. C

    B. pancreas
    C. right kidney
    D. transverse colon
    E. esophagus

33. The arterial supply of stomach comes from the
    A. left gastric artery
    B. splenic artery
    C. coeliac trunk
    D. superior mesenteric artery
    E. gastroduodenal artery

34. The pylorus of stomach
    A. is covered by the peritoneum only on its anterior aspect
    B. is indicated by the prepyloric vein
    C. is drained into superior mesenteric group of lymph nodes
    D. has only a physiological sphincter
    E. lies about an inch to the left of median plane

35. The stomach bed is formed by all the following structures *except* the
    A. body of the pancreas
    B. left kidney
    C. right kidney
    D. left suprarenal gland
    E. diaphragm

36. Which statement is *not* true regarding gastric nerves?
    A. Anterior gastric nerve mainly has right vagal fibres.
    B. Sympathetic fibres relax pyloric sphincter.
    C. Vagotomy reduces acid secretions.
    D. Sympathetic fibres come from T6-10 segments.

37. The part of stomach draining into pancreatico-splenic lymph nodes is
    A. adjoining to lesser curvature
    B. left part of Fundus and part adjoining to upper part of greater curvature.
    C. adjoining lower part of greater curvature.
    D. pyloric part.

Ans.   32. B   33. C   34. B   35. C   36. A   37. B

38. **Which of the following statements regarding stomach is *not* true?**
    A. Fundus lies above the level of cardiac orifice.
    B. Gastric canal runs along greater curvature.
    C. Is a common site for ulcers.
    D. Proximal and distal ends are more fixed parts.

39. **Sympathetic supply to stomach**
    A. comes from lumbar splanchnic nerves
    B. important for HCl secretion
    C. relaxes the pyloric sphincter
    D. important for vasomotor control

40. **Following statements about opening of stomach into duodenum are true *except***
    A. lies to the right of median plane.
    B. is called cardiac end
    C. is guarded by an anatomical sphincter
    D. lies at the level of first lumbar vertebra

41. **The first part of duodenum**
    A. terminates at fundus of gall bladder
    B. is the most mobile part of duodenum
    C. commences in subcostal plane
    D. supplied by superior mesenteric artery

42. **Duodenum is supplied by all the following arteries *except***
    A. common hepatic
    B. gastroduodenal
    C. splenic
    D. superior mesenteric

43. **First one inch of duodenum shows all the following features *except***
    A. is retroperitoneal
    B. forms lower boundary of epiploic foramen
    C. appears as duodenal cap in barium meal study
    D. gives attachment to lesser and greater omenta.

44. **Ligamentum teres represents obliterated**
    A. left umbilical vein

Ans. 38. B 39. D 40. B 41. B 42. C 43. A

B. right umbilical vein
C. right umbilical artery
D. peritoneal fold

45. The approximate length of duodenum is
   A. 15 cm
   B. 20 cm
   C. 25 cm
   D. 30 cm

46. Circular folds of the duodenum are absent in which part?
   A. First
   B. Second
   C. Third
   D. Fourth

47. Minor duodenal papilla marks the opening of
   A. bile duct
   B. major pancreatic duct
   C. accessory pancreatic duct
   D. hepato-pancreatic ampulla

48. All the following statements about third part of duodenum are true *except*
   A. it is the longest part
   B. is related above to head of pancreas
   C. is crossed anteriorly by superior mesenteric vessels
   D. is a common site for duodenal ulcer

49. The second part of the duodenum lies anterior to the
   A. inferior vena cava
   B. right kidney
   C. liver
   D. gall bladder
   E. transverse colon

50. The second part of duodenum
   A. lies on the right side of L2-L4 vertebrae
   B. is about 3 inches long
   C. is related anteriorly to the right colic flexure
   D. is completely covered by peritoneum anteriorly
   E. is supplied by the inferior pancreatico-duodenal artery only

Ans.   44. A   45. C   46. A   47. C   48. D   49. B   50. B

51. **The small intestine is supplied by the**
    A. coeliac trunk
    B. superior mesenteric artery
    C. inferior mesenteric artery
    D. coeliac trunk and superior mesenteric artery
    E. superior and inferior mesenteric arteries

52. **The colon can be distinguished by all the following features** *except*
    A. appendices epiploicae
    B. sacculations
    C. taenia coli
    D. no peritoneal covering

53. **The vermiform appendix**
    A. has three taenia coli
    B. always lies in the retrocaecal recess
    C. is supplied by a direct branch from the superior mesenteric artery
    D. opens into the caecum inferolateral to the opening of ileum
    E. is not covered by peritoneum at its tip

54. **The caecum**
    A. usually has a mesentery
    B. lies in the left iliac fossa
    C. lies on the iliacus and the quadratus lumborum muscles
    D. is supplied by ileocolic artery
    E. drains into the mesenteric lymph nodes

55. **Ascending colon has all the following features** *except*
    A. related laterally to right paracolic gutter
    B. is freely mobile
    C. supplied by ileocolic and right colic vessels
    D. lies on quadratus lumborum muscle

56. **All the following statements pertain to right colic flexure** *except*
    A. related to right lobe of liver
    B. supplied by superior mesenteric vessels
    C. supported by phrenico-colic ligament
    D. lies anterior to right kidney

Ans. 51. D 52. D 53. D 54. D 55. B 56. C

57. **All the following statements regarding left colic flexure are true** *except*
    A. lies higher than right colic flexure
    B. supplied by middle colic vessels
    C. supported by phrenico-colic ligament
    D. related to anterior end of spleen

58. **Transverse colon has all the following features** *except*
    A. forms a downward curve
    B. supplied by middle colic and left colic vessels
    C. is the shortest segment of colon
    D. is the most mobile segment of colon.

59. **Which part of large intestine makes S shaped course**
    A. ascending colon
    B. transverse colon
    C. splenic flexure
    D. sigmoid colon

60. **Transverse mesocolon**
    A. contains superior mesenteric vessels
    B. attached to head of pancreas
    C. attached to inferior border of body of pancreas
    D. lower layer is adherent to greater omentum

61. **Sigmoid mesocolon shows all the following features** *except*
    A. attachment is inverted V
    B. apex is near the division of right common iliac artery
    C. ureter descends behind the apex
    D. superior rectal vessels run along its right limb of attachment.

62. **Appendices epiploicae are absent from**
    A. caecum
    B. transverse colon
    C. sigmoid colon
    D. rectum

63. **The anal canal**
    A. length is 4 inches
    B. directed downwards and forwards
    C. anterior wall is smaller than posterior wall
    D. when empty lumen is a transverse slit.

Ans.   57. B   58. C   59. D   60. B   61. B   62. D   63. C

64. **All the following statements pertain to anal canal** *except*
    A. longitudinal folds of mucosa are present in the upper half.
    B. internal sphincter surrounds the entire length of anal canal.
    C. upper half is drained by superior rectal vein.
    D. the lining of lower half only is sensitive to pain.

65. **The venous radicals in anal columns are largest in all the following positions** *except*
    A. right anterior
    B. right posterior
    C. left lateral
    D. right lateral

66. **The external anal sphincter**
    A. has no bony attachment
    B. supplied by perineal branch of pudendal nerve
    C. composed of striated muscle
    D. located above the pelvic diaphragm

67. **The rectum**
    A. is a retroperitoneal structure
    B. shows usually three transverse folds
    C. is supported by Waldeyer's fascia
    D. malignancy may spread to sacral plexus
    E. shows all the above features

68. **The spleen**
    A. is covered by periotoneum only on its visceral surface
    B. is separated from the stomach by the lesser sac
    C. is related to both the left lung and the left pleura
    D. is drained into the left renal vein
    E. receives afferent lymph vessels like the lymph nodes

69. **The spleen**
    A. can be felt normally below the left costal margin
    B. destroys red blood corpuscles
    C. manufactures red blood corpuscles throughout life
    D. is related to the body of the pancreas
    E. is unaffected by the movements of respiration

70. **The pancreas**
    A. pours its secretions mainly through the minor duodenal papilla

Ans.   64. B   65. D   66. C   67. E   68. C   69. B

    B. is intraperitoneal organ

    C. is related posteriorly to the inferior vena cava and the aorta

    D. is supplied by the branches of the coeliac trunk only

    E. gives attachment to the mesentery of small intestine

71. The accessory pancreatic duct
    A. drains the body and tail of the pancreas
    B. opens into the minor duodenal papilla
    C. opens in common with the bile duct
    D. is surrounded by the sphincter of Oddi
    E. has none of the above properties

72. Upper border of body of pancreas is related to
    A. splenic vein
    B. splenic artery
    C. left gastric artery
    D. left renal vein

73. Pancreas is posteriorly related to all the following vessels *except*
    A. portal vein
    B. terminal part of renal veins
    C. inferior mesenteric artery
    D. superior mesenteric artery

74. The head of pancreas shows all the following features *except*
    A. it lies to the right of 2nd part of duodenum
    B. posteriorly related to inferior vena cava
    C. it is retroperitoneal
    D. anteriorly related to transverse colon

75. The quadrate lobe of liver is related to all the following structures *except*
    A. lower end of esophagus
    B. stomach pylorus
    C. first part duodenum
    D. transverse colon

76. All the following statements are true for the right lateral surface of liver *except*
    A. lies opposite 7-11 ribs in mid axillary line

Ans.   70. C   71. B   72. B   73. C   74. A   75. A

B. upper third is related to both lung and pleura
C. middle third is not related to pleura
D. lower third is separated from thoracic cage by diaphragm only.

77. **The gall-bladder shows all the following features *except***
A. consists of fundus, body and neck
B. fundus is covered with peritoneum all around
C. opens into cystic duct
D. average capacity is 100 ml

78. **The cystic duct**
A. has no valves
B. joins the common hepatic duct on its right side
C. shows Phrygian cap
D. is 3" long

79. **The caudate process of liver**
A. lies in front of the porta hepatis
B. lies in front of the superior recess of the lesser sac
C. forms the roof of the epiploic foramen
D. connects the caudate lobe with the rest of the left lobe of liver
E. is related to the second part of the duodenum

80. **The porta hepatis**
A. is a transverse fissure on the inferior surface of the left lobe of liver
B. transmits hepatic artery, hepatic vein and hepatic ducts
C. gives attachment to the lesser omentum
D. is a condensation of connective tissue
E. lies in front of the quadrate lobe

81. **The bare area of liver lies between the**
A. falciform ligament and the superior layer of coronary ligament
B. falciform ligament and the left triangular ligament
C. superior and the inferior layers of the coronary ligament
D. right and the left triangular ligaments

82. **The part of liver between the fissure for ligamentum venosum and the groove for inferior vena cava**
A. is not covered by peritoneum

Ans. 76. C 77. D 78. B 79. C 80. C 81. C

B. belongs to the anatomical left lobe of liver
C. functionally belongs to the right lobe of liver
D. is related to the esophagus
E. is related to the lesser sac and the diaphragm

83. **The gall bladder**
   A. lies to the right of the caudate lobe
   B. is completely covered by the peritoneum on its superior aspect
   C. is supplied by the cystic artery which is a branch of the right hepatic artery
   D. simply stores the bile juice
   E. secretes the bile juice

84. **The cystic duct**
   A. arises from the body of the gall bladder
   B. joins the right hepatic duct
   C. allows bile to flow only from gall bladder to the bile duct
   D. shows an outpouching called Hartman's pouch
   E. has a spiral valve in its interior

85. **The portal vein obstruction may result into all the following conditions *except* the**
   A. haemorrhoids
   B. esophageal varices
   C. caput medusae
   D. anal fistula

86. **All the following arise from the inferior mesenteric artery *except* the**
   A. left colic artery
   B. middle colic artery
   C. sigmoid arteries
   D. superior rectal artery

87. **The structures in the hilum of kidney are arranged from anterior to posterior side as**
   A. vein, ureter, artery
   B. artery, vein, ureter
   C. vein, artery, ureter
   D. ureter, artery, vein
   E. artery, ureter, vein

Ans.   82. E   83. C   84. E   85. D   86. B   87. C

88. The right kidney is related posteriorly to all the following structures *except* the
   A. diaphragm
   B. 11th rib
   C. transversus abdominis muscle
   D. psoas major muscle
   E. iliohypogastric nerve

89. Which of the following structures is related directly to the right kidney without the intervention of peritoneum?
   A. Liver
   B. Jejunum
   C. Duodenum
   D. Jejunal vessels

90. Which statement concerning right kidney is *not* correct?
   A. Enclosed in several facial sheaths
   B. Lies on iliacus muscle
   C. Related to branches of ventral primary ramus of first lumbar nerve
   D. Lies lower than left kidney

91. In diseases of right kidney pain is usually felt
   A. in the right hypochondrium
   B. at tip of right shoulder
   C. angle between right 12th rib and erecter spinae muscle
   D. around umbilicus

92. Renal fascia
   A. is also called true capsule
   B. both layers fuse inferiorly
   C. fuses medially with perivascular tissue
   D. encloses suprarenal gland in the same compartment as kidney.

93. Following statements regarding blood supply of kidney are true *except*
   A. renal artery is the branch of abdominal aorta
   B. accessory renal arteries are of common occurrence.
   C. accessory artery cannot cause ureteric obstruction
   D. ligation of accessory artery can result in infarction of the part supplied by that artery.

Ans.   88. B   89. C   90. B   91. C   92. C   93. C

94. **The ureter**
    A. enters the pelvis by crossing sacroiliac joint
    B. abdominal part should be mobilised laterally
    C. pelvic part should be mobilised medially
    D. measures about 15" in length

95. **Which surface of female urinary bladder is covered by peritoneum?**
    A. Base
    B. Superior
    C. Inferiolateral
    D. Anterior

96. **The smooth muscle fibres present around the neck of urinary bladder constitute**
    A. sphincter vesicae
    B. sphincter urethrae
    C. pubourethralis
    D. detrusor muscle

97. **The prostate gland**
    A. is covered by the peritoneum posteriorly
    B. lies between the medial borders of the two levator ani muscles
    C. cannot be felt through the rectum unless enlarged
    D. always undergoes hypertrophy in old age
    E. has a median lobe which lies between the ejaculatory ducts and the posterior surface of the prostate

98. **All the following features pertain to prostate gland *except***
    A. is conical in shape
    B. has five lobes
    C. prostatic venous plexus is between true and false capsule
    D. is an endocrine gland.

99. **The seminal vesicles have all the following features *except***
    A. sacculated, coiled tubules
    B. are supplied by inferior vesical and middle rectal vessels
    C. secretions are rich in fructose
    D. are normally palpable per rectum

Ans. 94. A   95. B   96. A   97. B   98. D   99. D

100. **The testes usually reach the scrotum in the**
    A. 7th month of intrauterine life
    B. 9th month of intrauterine life
    C. 1st year of life
    D. at puberty

101. **The deep dorsal vein of penis terminates into the**
    A. deep external pudendal vein
    B. prostatic venous plexus
    C. vesical venous plexus
    D. internal pudendal vein
    E. long saphenous vein

102. **The venous drainage of the right ovary is into the**
    A. internal iliac vein
    B. external iliac vein
    C. inferior vena cava
    D. right renal vein
    E. left renal vein

103. **Which is the narrowest part of fallopian tube?**
    A. Infundibulum
    B. Ampulla
    C. Isthmus
    D. Intramural part

104. **Which of the following is *not* a content of broad ligament?**
    A. Fallopian tube
    B. Uterine artery
    C. Ligament of ovary
    D. Ureter

105. **All the following are parts of broad ligament *except***
    A. infundibulo-pelvic ligament
    B. transverse cervical ligament
    C. mesosalpinx
    D. mesometrium

106. **All the following groups of lymphnodes are concerned with the drainage of the cervix uteri *except* the**
    A. internal iliac

Ans.   100. B   101. B   102. C   103. C   104. D   105. B

B. external iliac
C. sacral
D. deep inguinal
E. common iliac

107. The vagina
A. has an opening common to it and the urethra
B. lies in the axis of the pelvic inlet
C. meets the cervix of the uterus at approximately a right angle
D. has an anterior fornix deeper than the posterior fornix
E. is supplied by branches of the external iliac artery

108. The cavity of the body of the uterus
A. is large as compared to the thickness of its wall
B. is slit like in coronal section
C. shows mucosal folds
D. is constricted at its junction with the cavity of the cervix
E. shows none of the above properties

109. The most important factor in providing support to the uterus is the
A. round ligament of uterus
B. transverse ligament of cervix
C. recto-uterine fold of peritoneum
D. broad ligament
E. anteverted and anteflexed position of uterus

110. The isthmus of the uterus
A. is located above the level of the opening of the uterine tubes
B. lies adjacent to the external os
C. forms the lower uterine segment of the pregnant uterus
D. does not show any changes during menstrual cycle
E. has none of the above properties

111. The ischiorectal fossa
A. lies on either side of the rectum
B. allows for the distension of the rectum
C. has a lateral wall formed by the levator ani muscle and inferior fascia of the pelvic diaphragm

Ans.   106. D 107. C 108. D 109. B 110. C

  D. has pudendal canal in its lateral wall
  E. is crossed by the internal pudendal vessels from the lateral to the medial side

112. The pudendal nerve
  A. is the branch of the sacral plexus from S_1 to S_3 nerves
  B. leaves the pelvis through the lesser sciatic foramen
  C. crosses dorsal to sacrotuberous ligament
  D. terminates in the pudendal canal by diving into the perineal nerve and the dorsal nerve of the penis (or the clitoris)
  E. is purely a sensory nerve

113. The deep perineal pouch contains
  A. sphincter vesicae
  B. membranous urethra
  C. ejaculatory ducts
  D. root of penis
  E. pudendal nerve

114. The perineal body give attachment to
  A. levator ani muscles
  B. sphincter ani externus
  C. transverse perineal muscles
  D. all the above

115. The right suprarenal gland
  A. is oval in shape
  B. lies anterior to the inferior vena cava
  C. drains into the right renal vein
  D. is usually completely separated from the liver by the peritoneum
  E. is supplied by three arteries

116. The adrenal medulla
  A. secretes glucocorticoids
  B. secretes acetylcholine
  C. is mainly supplied by preganglonic sympathetic fibres
  D. is supplied by postganglionic sympathetic fibres only
  E. is essential for life

117. Left suprarenal gland
  A. is triangular in shape

Ans. 111. D 112. D 113. B 114. D 115. E 116. C

    B. lies posterior to lesser sac

    C. drains by three veins

    D. is supplied by single artery

118. **All the following statements are true about blood supply of suprarenal gland** *except*

    A. there are three arteries for each gland

    B. arteries enter the gland through hilus

    C. single vein leaves through hilus

    D. main artery is the direct branch of aorta

119. **Superior suprarenal artery is the branch of**

    A. aorta

    B. renal

    C. splenic

    D. inferior phrenic

120. **Regarding venous drainage of suprarenal gland**

    A. there are three veins on each side

    B. veins accompany the arteries

    C. right vein drains into inferior vena cava

    D. left vein drains into splenic vein

121. **All the following arteries are the direct branches from the abdominal aorta** *except* **the**

    A. superior mesenteric

    B. renal

    C. inferior phrenic

    D. inferior suprarenal

    E. gonadal

122. **All the following veins are the direct tributaries of the inferior vena cava** *except* **the**

    A. common iliac

    B. third lumbar

    C. left renal

    D. left gonadal

    E. right suprarenal

Ans. 117. B 118. B 119. D 120. C 121. D 122. D

123. All the following statements are true for the lumbar arteries *except* that they
   A. are usually four in number on each side
   B. pass under cover of the tendinous arches giving origin to the psoas major muscle
   C. supply only the structures forming the posterior abdominal wall
   D. also supply the spinal cord and cauda equina
   E. anastomose with other arteries of the abdominal walls

124. Which of the following nerves is *not* a branch of the sacral plexus?
   A. Superior gluteal
   B. Sciatic
   C. Pudendal
   D. Obturator
   E. Splanchnic

125. Which of the following arteries is *not* a branch of the internal iliac artery?
   A. Superior vesical
   B. Inferior vesical
   C. Ovarian
   D. Uterine
   E. Vaginal

126. The gastroduodenal artery is a branch of the
   A. coeliac trunk
   B. pancreaticoduodenal
   C. common hepatic
   D. superior mesenteric
   E. right gastric

127. The middle colic artery is a branch of the
   A. superior mesenteric artery
   B. coeliac trunk
   C. ileocolic
   D. right gastric
   E. inferior mesenteric

Ans. 123. C 124. D 125. C 126. C 127. A

128. **The pelvic splanchnic nerves**
    A. arise from upper three sacral nerves
    B. contain preganglionic sympathetic fibres
    C. contain postganglionic parasympathetic fibres
    D. supply motor fibres to he descending colon
    E. supply sensory fibres to the ascending colon

129. **Which of the following statements is *not* true for venous drainage of stomach?**
    A. Left gastroepiploic vein drains into splenic vein
    B. Right gastroepiploic vein drains into portal vein
    C. Left gastric vein communicates with esophageal veins
    D. Right gastric vein drains into hepatic vein

130. **Which of the following veins forms collateral channel in inferior vena caval obstruction?**
    A. Lateral thoracic vein
    B. Thoraco-epigastric vein
    C. Inferior epigastric vein
    D. Long thoracic vein

131. **Superior mesenteric vein**
    A. drains the hindgut
    B. terminates into inferior vena cava
    C. lies on the right side of superior mesenteric artery
    D. terminates at the level of L3 vertebra

132. **Cremasteric artery is the branch of**
    A. testicular artery
    B. superficial epigastric artery
    C. inferior epigastric artery
    D. internal pudenal artery

133. **Which statement regarding splenic artery is *not* true?**
    A. It is the branch of superior mesenteric artery
    B. It runs a tortuous course
    C. It runs along upper border of pancreas
    D. It reaches spleen through lieno-renal ligament

134. **Which statement regarding left gastric artery is *not* true?**
    A. It is the branch of coeliac trunk

Ans.   128. D 129. D 130. B 131. C 132. C 133. A

    B. It enters the lesser omentum at cardiac end of stomach

    C. It supplies lower end of esophagus

    D. Its proximal part often raises a fold of peritoneum called right gastropancreatic fold

135. **Which of the following statements about coeliac trunk is** *false*?

    A. It arises at L1 level

    B. It gives three branches

    C. It is the artery of foregut

    D. It is related to coeliac ganglion on either side

136. **Following statements are true for Inferior mesenteric artery** *except*

    A. it is an unpaired artery

    B. arises from aorta at L3 level

    C. related to corresponding vein on its left side

    D. continues as inferior rectal artery

137. **All the following are branches of superior mesenteric artery** *except*

    A. right colic

    B. ileocolic

    C. left colic

    D. jejunal

138. **Abdominal aorta bifurcates at the level of which lumbar vertebra?**

    A. Second

    B. Third

    C. Fourth

    D. Fifth

139. **Inferior vena cava is formed at the level of**

    A. third lumbar

    B. fourth lumbar

    C. fifth lumbar

    D. first sacral

140. **Short gastric branches reach the stomach through**

    A. lesser omentum

Ans. 134. D 135. A 136. D 137. C 138. C 139. C

B. gastrosplenic ligament
C. greater omentum
D. gastrophrenic ligament

141. **Which of the following is not a branch of posterior division of internal iliac artery?**
A. Superior gluteal
B. Iliolumbar
C. Median sacral
D. Lateral sacral

142. **All the following features pertain to right renal artery** *except*
A. it passes behind the inferior vena cava
B. it lies posterior to right renal vein
C. it lies in front of pelvis of ureter
D. it is shorter than left renal artery

143. **All the following structures cross anterior to aorta** *except*
A. left renal vein
B. root of mesentry
C. third part of duodenum
D. left lumbar veins

144. **Which of the following statements does** *not* **pertain to lumbar plexus?**
A. It is formed within quadratus lumborum muscle
B. Is formed by ventral rami of L1-L4
C. Gives rise to femoral and obturator nerves
D. Is connected to sacral plexus by nervous furcalis

145. **The lumbar sympathetic trunk**
A. usually has five ganglia
B. all lumbar splanchnic nerves join superior hypogastric plexus
C. enters abdomen behind lateral arcuate ligament
D. runs along medial border of psoas major

146. **Pelvic part of sympathetic trunk**
A. runs along lateral side of pelvic sacral foramina
B. caudally the two trunks join to form ganglion impar
C. ganglion impar lies in front of lower end of sacrum
D. gives rise to pelvic splanchnic nerves

Ans.   140. B 141. C 142. D 143. D 144. A 145. D 146. B

147.   Cancer Metastasis from which of the following organs will
       involve lungs at relatively earlier stage?
       A.   Caecum
       B.   Stomach
       C.   Duodenum
       D.   Kidney

148.   Ligation of common hepatic artery below the origin of
       gastroduodenal artery will allow blood supply to liver to be
       carried by which of the following anastomosis?
       A.   Short gastric and left gastric
       B.   Right and left gastroepiploic
       C.   Right and left gastric
       D.   Right and left hepatic

149.   During surgery in the region of gall bladder, excess
       haemorrhage can be controlled by compressing
       A.   right hepatic artery at origin
       B.   right branch of portal vein
       C.   right hepatic vein
       D.   both common hepatic artery and portal vein in free margin of
            lesser omentum

150.   Rupture of urethra in superficial perineal pouch leads to
       extravasation of urine into all the following areas *except*
       A.   thigh
       B.   scrotum
       C.   penis
       D.   anterior abdominal wall

Directions: For each of the incomplete statements or questions below, one
or more completions or answers is correct. Select
       A.   if one 1,2 and 3 are correct;
       B.   if only 1 and 3 are correct;
       C.   if only 2 and 4 are correct;
       D.   if only 4 is correct;
       E.   if all are correct.

---

151.   **The inlet of the pelvis**
       1.   is formed posteriorly by the promontory of sacrum
       2.   makes an angle of about 55° with the horizontal

Ans.   147. D 148. B 149. D 150. A

3. is about 13.0 cm transversely in females
4. is heart shaped in females

152. The sacrum
1. has a promontory at the junction of the bodies of the first and second sacral vertebrae
2. is more curved in males
3. is related anteriorly to the rectum and anal canal
4. is connected to ilium and ischium by ligaments

153. The ischial spine
1. gives attachment to the levator ani and coccygeus muscles
2. is crossed externally by the pudendal nerve
3. can be felt through the vagina
4. can not be felt through the rectum

154. The transpyloric plane
1. lies at the level of the first lumbar vertebra
2. cuts the costal margin at the tip of the 9th costal cartilage
3. is an important landmark for dividing the abdomen into different areas
4. lies midway between the suprasternal notch and the upper border of pubic symphysis

155. The transversus abdominis muscle
1. lies between the internal and external oblique muscles of abdomen
2. lies immediately behind the rectus abdominis muscle throughout
3. forms cremaster muscle
4. takes part in the formation of conjoint tendon

156. The inguinal canal
1. is about 4 cm long
2. lies parallel to the inguinal ligament
3. is formed anteriorly by the aponeurosis of the external oblique muscle and fleshy fibres of the internal oblique muscle
4. is wider in the females

157. The spermatic cord contains the
1. ductus deferens
2. testicular artery

Ans.   151. A 152. D 153. B 154. E 155. D 156. A

3. pampiniform plexus of veins
4. ilioinguinal nerve

158. The superficial inguinal ring
1. is an opening in the aponeurosis of internal oblique muscle
2. lies superomedial to the pubic crest
3. transmits the spermatic cord and the iliohypogastric nerve in males
4. is strengthened by the conjoint tendon posteriorly

159. The linea alba
1. extends from the xiphoid process to the pubic symphysis
2. is formed by the decussation of aponeurotic fibres of the external oblique and the internal oblique muscles only
3. is relatively avascular
4. is broad in its infraumblical part

160. The cremaster muscle
1. is derived from the transversus abdominis muscle
2. lies between the external and the internal spermatic fascia
3. is supplied by the ilioinguinal nerve
4. retracts the testis

161. The boundaries of the Hasselbach's triangle include the
1. inferior epigastric vessels
2. medial border of the rectus abdominis muscle
3. inguinal ligament
4. median umbilical fold

162. The direct inguinal hernia
1. is usually congenital
2. lies medial to the inferior epigastric vessels
3. enters directly through the deep inguinal ring
4. does not have internal spermatic fascia as one of its coverings

163. The diaphragm
1. is tendinous in its peripheral part and muscular in its central part
2. is related inferiorly to the stomach and the spleen
3. relaxes in all expulsive acts like vomiting, sneezing, crying etc.
4. shows an excursion of about 6-10 cm in deep inspiration

Ans.   157. A 158. D 159. B 160. C 161. B 162. C 163. C

164. Which of the following statements are true about the diaphragm?
1. Contraction of diaphragm assists in venous return to the heart
2. Contraction of left crus help in preventing regurgitation of food from stomach into the esophagus
3. On contraction, the central tendon descends and the intrathoracic pressure falls
4. The level of diaphragm is unaffected by posture or large meal

165. The levator ani muscle arises from the
1. pelvic surface of the superior ramus of pubis
2. obturator fascia
3. obturator membrane
4. ischial spine

166. The levator ani muscle
1. is related superiorly to the urinary bladder, the prostate and the rectum
2. forms the medial wall of the ischiorectal fossa
3. posteriorly is related to coccygeus muscle
4. has a medial border which is separated from the medial border of the other levator ani by a gap

167. The urogenital diaphragm
1. consists of the sphincter urethrae and superficial transversus perinei muscles
2. is pierced by the prostatic part of urethra
3. is supplied by spinal segments, S1, S2 and S3
4. lies below the pelvic diaphragm

168. The superficial perineal pouch
1. lies between the perineal membrane and the membranous layer of superficial fascia of perineum
2. is a closed space
3. contains the root of penis (or clitoris)
4. gives passage to the membranous urethra

169. The perineal body
1. lies between the anal canal and the vagina
2. is a fibromuscular structure

Ans.   164. B   165. C   166. E   167. D   168. B

3. may get torn during parturition
4. supports the vagina

170. The stomach
1. gives attachment to the lesser omentum along its lesser curvature
2. lies behind the lesser sac
3. moves with respiration
4. does not extend above the level of the costal margin

171. The venous drainage of the stomach is into the
1. portal vein
2. inferior mesenteric vein
3. superior mesenteric vein
4. inferior vena cava

172. The duodenum
1. is entirely retroperitoneal
2. is related posteriorly to the right and left ureters
3. is 12 inches long
4. shows the opening of the bile duct about 10 cm from the pyloroduodenal junction

173. The jejunum can be distinguished from the ileum by the presence of
1. long vasa recta
2. less fat in the mesentery
3. fewer arterial arcades
4. fewer number of circular folds

174. The Meckel's diverticulum
1. is a remnant of allantois
2. occurs on the mesenteric border of the ileum
3. is always connected to the umbilicus by a fibrous cordlike structure
4. often has gastric mucosa in its lining

175. The left colic flexure
1. lies at a level lower than that of the right colic flexure
2. is supplied by the middle colic artery

Ans. 169. E 170. B 171. B 172. D 173. A 174. D

    3. is related to the spleen directly without the intervention of peritoneum

    4. is supplied by parasympathetic fibres from sacral outflow

176. The structures that can be felt through the anterior wall of the rectum are the
1. bulb of penis
2. prostate
3. cervix uteri
4. ureters

177. The blood supply to the rectum comes from the
1. median sacral artery
2. superior rectal artery
3. middle rectal artery
4. inferior rectal artery

178. The rectum
1. runs a straight course through the pelvis
2. has a dilated upper part called the ampulla
3. is related posteriorly to the lower four pieces of sacrum and the coccyx
4. forms the posterior wall of pouch of Douglas

179. The McBurney's point is
1. the junction of the lateral 2/3 and medial 1/3 of the line joining the anterior superior iliac spine and the umbilicus
2. the point of maximum tenderness in appendicitis
3. the point of maximum tenderness in the inflammation of the gall bladder
4. is used for making skin incision for appendicectomy

180. The spleen
1. is an intraperitoneal organ
2. moves with respiration
3. lies in the long axis of the 10th rib
4. is connected to the right kidney by the lieno-renal ligament

181. The liver
1. receives blood from the hepatic artery only
2. drains into the portal vein

Ans.   175. D 176. A 177. A 178. D 179. C 180. A

3. is normally palpable in the right hypochondrium
4. moves with respiration

182. The bile duct
1. is about 7.5 cm long
2. is about 1 cm wide
3. lies in the free margin of the lesser omentum
4. is related to the gastroduodenal artery behind the head of the pancreas

183. The bile duct
1. Formed by union of right and left hepatic ducts
2. Opens into first part of duodenum
3. Related laterally to hepatic artery
4. Related posteriorly to portal vein

184. The portal vein
1. is formed behind the neck of the pancreas
2. lies in the anterior wall of the epiploic foramen
3. receives blood from the abdominal part of the gastrointestinal tract
4. is formed by the union of the splenic and the inferior mesenteric veins

185. The body of the pancreas
1. crosses the posterior abdominal wall in a horizontal plane
2. gives attachment to the transverse mesocolon
3. is separated from the stomach by the greater sac
4. has splenic artery along its upper border

186. The blood supply to pancreas comes from
1. splenic artery
2. left gastroepiploic artery
3. superior mesenteric artery
4. hepatic artery proper

187. The left kidney
1. lies higher than the right kidney
2. is separated from the stomach by the greater sac
3. drains into the lateral aortic lymph nodes
4. receives blood from the left suprarenal gland

Ans. 181. D 182. A 183. D 184. A 185. C 186. B 187. B

188. The left kidney
1. is related anteriorly to the fourth part of the duodenum
2. has five vascular segments
3. is related to the left lung and pleura
4. is surrounded by the renal fascia which also encloses the left suprarenal gland

189. The ureter
1. has two third of its length in the abdomen
2. shows a constriction at the pelviureteric junction
3. lies along the bases of the transverse processes of the lumbar vertebrae
4. is supplied by the inferior vesical artery in its pelvic part

190. The ureter in the female
1. forms the anterior boundary of the ovarian fossa
2. crosses above the uterine artery
3. lies in close apposition to the cervix uteri
4. passes slightly above the lateral fornix of vagina

191. The arterial supply of the left ureter comes from
1. gonadal artery
2. renal artery
3. inferior vesical artery
4. inferior mesenteric artery

192. The urinary bladder
1. is covered by peritoneum on its inferolateral surfaces
2. shows in its interior a relatively pinkish area called trigone
3. is supplied by parasympathetic fibres through the vagus nerve
4. when full rises above the pelvic inlet

193. Which of the following statements are true for the urinary bladder?
1. It lies at the same level in the infants and the adults
2. It shows an elevation called the uvula due to the median lobe of the prostate gland
3. The internal urethral meatus rises as the bladder fills up
4. Its mucous coat shows folds all over except the region of trigone

Ans.   188. C   189. C   190. D   191. A   192. D   193. C

194. **The sphincters under voluntary control are**
     1. sphincter urethrae
     2. sphincter vesicae
     3. sphincter ani externus
     4. sphincter ani internus

195. **The prostate**
     1. lies on the urogenital diaphragm
     2. is transversed by the ductus deferens
     3. can be felt through the rectum
     4. lies behind the base of urinary bladder

196. **The prostatic venous plexus communicates with the**
     1. vesical venous plexus
     2. vertebral venous plexus
     3. internal iliac vein
     4. external iliac vein

197. **The prostatic urethra**
     1. lies nearer to the posterior surface of the prostate
     2. shows a crest along its anterior wall
     3. is surrounded by the sphincter urethrae
     4. shows openings of the ejaculatory ducts

198. **The membranous urethra**
     1. has membranous walls
     2. is the least dilatable part of the urethra
     3. lies in the superficial perineal pouch
     4. is surrounded by the sphincter urethrae

199. **The seminal vesicles**
     1. lie between the base of the urinary bladder and the rectum
     2. pour their secretions directly into the prostatic urethra
     3. lie lateral to the ductus deferens
     4. have fibromuscular stroma

200. **The ductus deferens**
     1. is about 18 cm long
     2. joins the duct of the seminal vesicle to form the ejaculatory duct

Ans.   194. B   195. B   196. A   197. D   198. C   199. B

3. is ligated in the operation of vasectomy
4. is usually supplied by a branch from the superior vesical artery

201. The testis
1. is completely enclosed in the tunica vaginalis
2. is related to the epididymis along its posterior border
3. is supplied by the testicular artery which is a branch of the internal iliac artery
4. drains into lateral aortic lymph nodes

202. The ovary
1. lies on the psoas major muscle
2. is connected to the uterus by the round ligament
3. is attached to anterior layer of broad ligament
4. is covered by the peritoneum all around except along its anterior border

203. The fallopian tube
1. lies in the medial 4/5 part of the free border of the broad ligament
2. has an ampulla which is its most distensible part
3. pierces the peritoneum at its lateral end
4. is ligated in the family planning operation in females

204. The uterus
1. lies anterior to the urinary bladder
2. has a fundus which is covered by peritoneum all around
3. is supplied by the uterine artery which first reaches it near its fundus
4. normally is anteverted and anteflexed

205. The cervix
1. has an upper part called the isthmus
2. has an intravaginal part covered by the stratified squamous epithelium
3. is not covered with the peritoneum anteriorly
4. opens into the vagina through the internal os

206. The vagina
1. has an anterior wall which is longer than the posterior wall
2. is covered by the peritoneum in the region of posterior fornix only

Ans.   200. E 201. C 202. D 203. E 204. C 205. A

3. is related to the perineal body anteriorly
4. is related to the base of the urinary bladder and urethra anteriorly

207. The perineum is supplied by the
1. pudendal nerve
2. inferior gluteal nerve
3. posterior cutaneous nerve of thigh
4. medial cutaneous nerve of thigh

208. The left suprarenal gland
1. is semilunar in shape
2. lies on the left crus of the diaphragm
3. forms part of the stomach bed
4. drains into the left renal vein

209. The lumbar plexus
1. receives contribution from all the lumbar nerves
2. is formed within the substance of the psoas major muscle
3. gives rise to the femoral nerve which emerges at the medial border of the psoas major
4. gives off the obturator nerve from ventral division of L2-L4 nerves

210. The abdominal aorta
1. bifurcates at the level of fourth lumbar vertebra
2. lies directly on the vertebral column
3. is crossed anteriorly by the left renal vein just below the origin of the superior mesenteric artery
4. is crossed by the first and third parts of the duodenum

211. The inferior vena cava
1. is formed at the level of fourth lumbar vertebra
2. lies behind the liver and the head of the pancreas
3. is crossed anteriorly by the right renal artery
4. is separated from the first part of the duodenum by the portal vein

212. The superior mesenteric artery
1. supplies the whole of the small intestine
2. origin lies between the splenic and the left renal veins

Ans. 206. C 207. B 208. E 209. C 210. A 211. C

    3. descends posterior to the uncinate process of pancreas

    4. lies in the root of the mesentery

213. The inferior mesenteric vein

    1. terminates in the splenic vein

    2. lies lateral to the corresponding artery

    3. often lies in the paraduodenal fold of peritoneum

    4. is the continuation of the middle rectal vein

214. The sacral plexus

    1. is formed by the dorsal rami of L4-S3 nerves

    2. is formed in front of the piriformis muscle

    3. lies anterior to the internal iliac vessels

    4. can be compressed by the fetal head

215. The marginal artery of the large intestine is formed by the branches of the

    1. coeliac trunk

    2. superior mesenteric artery

    3. gastroduodenal artery

    4. inferior mesenteric artery

216. The posterior vagal trunk

    1. contains fibres predominantly from the left vagus nerve

    2. gives a branch to the coeliac plexus

    3. contains postganglionic parasympathetic fibres

    4. gives gastric branches to supply mainly the postero-inferior surface of the stomach

217. In relation to the nerve supply of the urinary bladder

    1. the parasympathetic supply comes through the vagus nerve

    2. the sympathetic innervation is through the inferior hypogastric plexus

    3. the parasympathetic fibres synapse with neurons scattered in hypogastric plexuses

    4. the sympathetic fibres have preganglionic neurons located in spinal segments T10-L2.

218. In relation to the nerve supply of the urinary bladder

    1. the parasympathetic fibres are motor to the detrusor muscle

---

Ans.   212. C 213. A 214. C 215. C 216. C 217. C

2. the sympathetic fibres are inhibitory to the sphincter vesicae
3. the pain fibres are carried by both the sympathetic and parasympathetic fibres
4. the sensation of distension and pain are carried by the posterior column tracts in the spinal cord

219. In relation to the lymphatic drainage of rectum and anal canal
1. upper half of rectum drains into para rectal and inferior mesenteric lymph nodes
2. lower half of rectum drains into internal iliac lymph nodes
3. anal canal above the mucocutaneous junction drains into internal iliac lymph nodes
4. anal canal below the mucocutaneous junction drains into deep inguinal lymph nodes

220. The lymph nodes draining the body of the uterus include
1. lateral aortic
2. internal iliac
3. superficial inguinal
4. sacral

Directions: Each question consists of an assertion and a reason. Responses should be choosen as follows:
A. if the assertion and reason are true statements and the reason is a correct explanation of the assertion;
B. if the assertion and reason are true statements but the reason is not a correct explanation of the assertion;
C. if the assertion is true but the reason is a false statement;
D. if the assertion is false but the reason is a true statement;
E. if both assertion and reason are false statements.

---

221. The skin around the umbilicus is supplied by the fourth lumbar nerve
Because
the umbilicus usually lies at the level of fourth lumbar vertebra

---

Ans. 218. B 219. A 220. E 221. D

222. The lateral part of the anterior wall of inguinal canal is strengthened by the presence of internal oblique muscle
Because
the posterior wall of the inguinal canal is weakened in this region by the presence of the superficial inguinal ring

223. In the indirect inguinal hernia, the coverings include internal spermatic fiscia
Because
The indirect hernia enters the inguinal canal through the deep inguinal ring

224. To relieve the strangulation in the case of indirect inguinal hernia the deep inguinal ring should not be enlarged medially
Because
the inferior epigastric vessels lie medial to the deep inguinal ring

225. The tendinous intersections in the rectus abdominis muscle make the muscle stronger
Because
the intersections are attached to the anterior rectus sheath only

226. Scratching the skin on the medial side of the upper part of the thigh results in retraction of the testis in the abdomen
Because
the testis originally develops in the abdomen

227. The incidence of inguinal hernia is more in females
Because
the pelvis is wider in females

228. The stomach is supplied by the coeliac trunk
Because
it develops from the foregut

229. Stomach contents normally do not regurgitate into the esophagus
Because
the circular muscle is thickened to form a sphincter at the cardio-esophageal junction

---

Ans.   222. C 223. A 224. A 225. B 226. B 227. D 228. A 229.C

230.   **The anterior surface of stomach receives fibres mainly from the right vagal trunk**

Because

the anterior surface represents the original right surface of stomach prior to rotation

231.   **The terminal part of the ileum is supplied by branches of the ileocolic artery**

Because

it opens into the junction of the caecum and the ascending colon

232.   **The splenic artery reaches the spleen through the gastrosplenic ligament**

Because

the gastroplenic ligament is a part of the original dorsal mesogastrium

233.   **The splenic flexure of the colon is supplied by the splenic artery**

Because

this flexure is closely related to the spleen

234.   **The spleen moves with respiration**

Because

it is connected to the diaphragm by a fold of peritoneum

235.   **In appendicitis the pain is referred to umbilical region**

Because

The appendix develops from the midgut which herniates through the umbilical opening during intrauterine life

236.   **The ascending colon is less mobile**

Because

it has a short mesentery

237.   **The lesions above the pectinate line of anal canal are not very painful**

Because

this region is supplied by the autonomic nerves

Ans.   230. E   231. B   232. D   233. D   234. C   235. B   236. E   237. A

238. **The ligation of the middle colic artery will cut off blood supply to the transverse colon**
Because
this is the main artery supplying the transverse colon

239. **The pancreas is highly mobile**
Because
it gives attachment to the transverse mesocolon.

240. **The left kidney is related to both the left lung and the left pleura**
Because
it lies higher than the right kidney

241. **The suprarenal gland lies within the renal fascia**
Because
it develops in close relation to the kidney

242. **The urinary bladder cannot be approached extra-peritoneally**
Because
the anterior abdominal wall is lined by the parietal peritoneum

243. **The fallopian tube pierces the peritoneum**
Because
the ova are liberated into the peritoneal cavity

244. **The lymphatic drainage of testis is into the superficial inguinal lymph nodes**
Because
the scrotal sac drains into this group of lymph nodes

245. **It is not possible to drain the pouch of Douglas through the vagina**
Because
the vagina is not at all covered by peritoneum

246. **The cervix uteri can be visualised through the vagina**
Because
the cervix lies in the axis of the vagina

Ans.   238.D 239.D 240.D 241.C 242.D 243.A 244.D 245. E 246.C

247. **The enlarged seminal vesicles can be felt through the rectum**
Because
they lie in direct relation to the anterior wall of the rectum

248. **Pain arising from the hollow viscera is usually poorly localised**
Because
the visceral pain fibres are carried by the autonomic nerves

249. **On barium meal examination the most proximal part of the duodenum has a smooth appearance**
Because
there are no villi in this part of the duodenum

250. **The division of anorectal ring can lead to incontinence of faeces**
Because
the puborectalis muscle is responsible for maintaining the perineal flexure of rectum.

Ans. 247. A 248. A 249. C 250. A

PART- II

HISTOLOGY

CHAPTER 6

Histology

Directions: Each of the incomplete statements or questions below is followed by four or five suggested completions or answers. Select the one which is BEST in each case.

1. **Which of the following statements is true for the unit of measurement in microscopy?**
   A. One micrometer is 1/100 of a millimeter
   B. One nanometer is 1/10000 of a micron
   C. One nanometer is 1/1000 of a millimeter
   D. One micrometer is 1/1000 of a millimeter

2. **Which of the following cells does *not* have a nucleus?**
   A. Neuron   B. Red blood cell
   C. White blood cell   D. Macrophage
   E. Fibrocyte

3. **Under the electron microscope a centriole consists of**
   A. nine pairs of tubules
   B. nine pairs of outer tubules and one pair of central tubules
   C. nine groups of tubules, each group having three microtubules
   D. nine groups of three microtubules each, arranged around a central pair of microtubules

4. **The cell organelle responsible for intracellular digestion of phagocytosed material is the**
   A. golgi apparatus   B. centrosome
   C. lysosome   D. mitochondrion
   E. ribosome

5. **Transitional epithelium has all the following features *except***
   A. consists of 4-6 layers of cells

Ans.   1. D   2. B   3. C   4. C

B. superficial cells are umbrella shaped
C. deepest layer is impermeable to urine
D. it is easily stretchable

6. **The transitional epithelium is present in the**
   A. ductus deferens
   B. ureter
   C. terminal part of urethra
   D. seminal vesicle
   E. vagina

7. **Which type of gland is a sebaceous gland?**
   A. Apocrine
   B. Holocrine
   C. Merocrine
   D. Endocrine
   E. None of the above

8. **Which of the following cells is *not* a connective tissue cell?**
   A. Macrophage
   B. Plasma cell
   C. Pericyte
   D. Mast cell
   E. Adipose cell

9. **The elastic cartilage is present in all the following sites *except* the**
   A. pinna
   B. epiglottis
   C. trachea
   D. auditory tube
   E. corniculate cartilage of larynx

10. **All the following statements pertain to hyaline cartilage *except***
    A. it has pearly bluish translucent appearance
    B. all temporary cartilages are of hyaline variety
    C. matrix is typically basophillic and homogenous
    D. cell nests are seen at periphery

Ans.   5. C   6. B   7. B   8. C   9. C   10. D

11. **Microanatomy of compact bone shows all the following features *except***
    A. circumferential lamellae under the periosteum
    B. concentric lamellae around Haversian canal
    C. lacunae connected with each other and Haversian canal through canaliculi
    D. vertically running Volkman's canals.

12. **Which of the following is a content of lacunae in the bone?**
    A. Osteoblast
    B. Osteocyte
    C. Osteoclast
    D. Osteogenic cell

13. **Which of the following is not part of Haversian system?**
    A. Haversian canal
    B. Concentric lamellae
    C. Neurovascular bundle
    D. Lymph vessels

14. **Which of the following is *not* a bone cell?**
    A. Osteophyte
    B. Osteoblast
    C. Osteoclast
    D. Osteocyte

15. **The osteoclast**
    A. is almost equal in size to an osteoblast
    B. has a single large nucleus
    C. is rich in rough endoplasmic reticulum
    D. is concerned with absorption of bone
    E. is concerned with deposition of bone

16. **The skeletal muscle fibre can be differentiated from the smooth muscle fibre by all the following features *except* that**
    A. it is cylindrical in shape
    B. it shows alternate light and dark bands
    C. it has a single oval nucleus
    D. its nuclei are situated at the periphery
    E. each fibre is innervated by a branch of an axon

Ans.   11. D   12. B   13. D   14. A   15. D   16. C

17. **When a skeletal muscle fibre contracts there is a shortening of the**
    A. A bands
    B. I bands
    C. H bands
    D. A bands and I bands
    E. I bands and H bands

18. **The Nissl substance is**
    A. present only in the perinuclear region in the neuron
    B. present in the region of axon hillock
    C. not present in the dendrites
    D. composed of neurofibrils
    E. prominent in the alpha neurons of the spinal cord

19. **Meiosis is characterised by all the following features** *except* **that**
    A. it consists of two successive divisions
    B. DNA duplication does not occur
    C. crossing over occurs between homologous chromosomes
    D. in the daughter cells, the chromosome number is reduced to half
    E. the daughter cells are not identical

20. **The epithelial tissue has all the following features** *except* **that**
    A. all the cells rest on a basement membrane
    B. the cells are separated by minimum of intercellular substance
    C. the free surface of epithelial cells may show microvilli if the cells have absorptive function
    D. it is generally devoid of blood vessels
    E. it shows considerable capacity or repair after damage

The mast cells are believed to release
    A. heparin
    B. histamine
    C. serotonin
    D. all the above
    E. none of the above

Ans. 17. E   18. E   19. B   20. A 21. D

22. **The sinusoids are present in all the following organs** *except*
    A. liver
    B. spleen
    C. adenohypophysis
    D. thyroid
    E. parathyroid

23. **Which of the following organs does** *not* **show a division into cortex and medulla?**
    A. Lymph node
    B. Thymus
    C. Spleen
    D. Suprarenal
    E. Kidney

24. **The gland which undergoes involution with age is**
    A. pancreas
    B. thymus
    C. thyroid
    D. suprarenal
    E. hypophysis cerebri

25. **The lymphoid nodules are** *not* **seen in the**
    A. lymph node
    B. thymus
    C. spleen
    D. tonsil
    E. appendix

26. **All the following features pertain to microscopic structure of lymph node** *except*
    A. shows cortex and medulla
    B. there is subcapsular lymph sinus
    C. lymphoid nodules may show germinal centre
    D. lymphoid nodules are present in medulla

27. **Palatine tonsil shows all the following features** *except*
    A. collection of lymphoid tissue
    B. there is no cortex and medulla
    C. surface shows crypts covered by stratified squamous epithelium
    D. shows Hassal's corpuscles

Ans.   22. D   23. C   24. B   25. B   26. D   27. D

28. **Which of the following statements is correct for circulation through spleen?**
   A. Penicilli are surrounded by lymphoid tissue
   B. Penicilli open into sinusoids
   C. Sinusoids comprise high proportion of red pulp.
   D. Circulation is closed type as in other organs

29. **Which of the following features is true for tongue?**
   A. It is covered by stratified columnar epithelium
   B. Its musculature is made up of smooth muscle fibres arranged in various directions
   C. The taste buds are confined to the vallate papillae
   D. The pharyngeal surface is devoid of papillae but shows collections of lymphoid tissue
   E. There are no glands in its substance

30. **All the following features pertain to microanatomy of tongue** *except*
   A. surface covered by epithelial cells having microvilli
   B. surface shows numerous papillae
   C. skeletal muscle arranged in all directions
   D. taste buds present on its inferior surface

31. **Which of the following glands has serous demilunes?**
   A. Parotid gland
   B. Submandibular gland
   C. Lacrimal gland
   D. Pancreas gland

32. **Mucus secreting glands in submucosa are seen in which of the following?**
   A. Gall bladder
   B. Pyloric part of stomach
   C. Duodenum
   D. Colon

33. **A section shows closely packed small acini with numerous ducts scattered between them. The cells lining the acini are darkly stained and have spherical nuclei towards the base. The section is through the**
   A. sublingual salivary gland

Ans. 28. C   29. D   30. A   31. B   32. C

   B.   submandibular salivary gland
   C.   parotid gland
   D.   pancreas
   E.   lacrimal gland

34. The goblet cells are *not* present in the
   A.   stomach
   B.   small intestine
   C.   large intestine
   D.   trachea
   E.   bronchi

35. The main gastric glands
   A.   are present only in the body of the stomach
   B.   are coiled tubular glands
   C.   contain chief cells which are more numerous than the oxyntic cells
   D.   extend into the submucosa
   E.   have none of the above properties

36. The most characteristic histological feature of the duodenum is the presence of
   A.   numerous large villi
   B.   prominent circular folds
   C.   glands of Brunner in the submucosa
   D.   paneth cells in the crypts of Lieberkuhn
   E.   numerous goblet cells

37. The large intestine has all the following features *except*
   A.   numerous goblet cells
   B.   only a few villi
   C.   longitudinal muscle layer in the form of three bands
   D.   no glands in the submucosa
   E.   numerous intestinal glands in the lamina propria

38. All the statements regarding peritoneum are true *except*
   A.   free surface is lined by simple cuboidal epithelium
   B.   parietal peritoneum is pain sensitive
   C.   provides large absorptive surface
   D.   allows movement of viscera without friction

Ans.   33. C   34. A   35. C   36. C   37. B   38. A

39. **All the following statements regarding paneth cells are true except**
    A. present in deeper parts of crypts of Lieberkuhn
    B. present in both small and large intestine
    C. rich in Zinc
    D. secrete digestive enzymes

40. **Which of the following glands has fibromuscular stroma?**
    A. Pancreas
    B. Prostate
    C. Parotid
    D. Pituitary

41. **Which of the following organs has both smooth and skeletal muscle is its muscle coat?**
    A. Colon
    B. Ileum
    C. Stomach
    D. Esophagus

42. **The pyloric part of stomach**
    A. outer longitudinal layer is broken into three longitudinal bands
    B. submucosa contains pyloric glands
    C. pyloric glands are coiled, tubular, mucus secreting glands
    D. gastric pits are shallow

43. **All the following features pertain to intrahepatic biliary apparatus except**
    A. hepatocytes are polyhedral cells that produce bile
    B. bile canaliculi have walls made of modified surface of hepatocytes
    C. bile canaliculi surround all surfaces of hepatocytes
    D. bile ductules lie in portal triads

44. **The following features pertain to microanatomy of liver except**
    A. hepatic lobule has hepatic vein in the centre
    B. portal lobule is supplied by one portal triad
    C. liver acinus is the tissue supplied by a terminal branch of hepatic artery
    D. adjacent portal lobules are separated by connective tissue

Ans.   39. B   40. B   41. D   42. C   43. C   44. D

45. **Smooth muscle fibres**
    A. they are cylindrical in shape
    B. they are mononucleated
    C. nucleus is located just under the sarcolemna
    D. fibres are connected by intercalated discs

46. **The B-cells of pancreas secrete**
    A. glucagon
    B. somatostatin
    C. insulin
    D. amylase
    E. pancreatic polypeptide

47. **The part of a nephron lined by cells showing microvilli is the**
    A. Bowman's capsule
    B. proximal convoluted tubule
    C. loop of Henle
    D. distal convoluted tubule
    E. collecting ducts

48. **The number of nephrons in one kidney is approximately**
    A. ten thousand
    B. fifty thousand
    C. one million
    D. five million
    E. ten million

49. **All the following statements regarding nephron are true** *except*
    A. lined by simple epithelium throughout
    B. active resorption occurs in proximal convoluted tubule
    C. cells of proximal tubule are under the action of antidiuretic hormone
    D. mesangial cells present in relation to glomerulus are phagocytic

50. **All the following statements pertaining to microanatomy of urinary bladder are true** *except*
    A. it is lined by transitional epithelium except in the region of trigone
    B. mucosa is thrown into folds except over trigone
    C. there is no submucosa
    D. muscle coat has three indistinct layers

Ans.   45. B   46. C   47. B   48. C   49. C   50. A

51. **The number of seminiferous tubules in one testis is approximately**
    A. 100
    B. 500
    C. 5,000
    D. 10,000
    E. 1,00,000

52. **The interstitial cells of testis**
    A. located in the wall of seminiferous tubules
    B. activity is controlled by growth stimulating hormone of anterior pituitary
    C. form part of blood testis barrier
    D. absent in cryptorchid testis

53. **The stroma is fibromuscular in the**
    A. seminal vesicles
    B. testis
    C. epididymis
    D. prostate
    E. thyroid

54. **A section shows profiles of tubules of various shapes. The tubules do *not* have a distinct lumen and are lined by several layers of cells of various sizes. The section is through the**
    A. epididymis
    B. testis
    C. seminal vesicle
    D. thyroid
    E. prostate

55. **Which of the following statements is true about the structure of the parathyroid gland?**
    A. It consists of two types of cells and ducts
    B. The chief cells are smaller in size and more numerous than the oxyphil cells
    C. The chief cells are deeply eosinophillic
    D. The oxyphil cells secrete parathormone
    E. The number of oxyphil cells decreases with age

Ans.   51. B   52. D   53. D   54. B   55. B

56. **The corpora arenacea are seen in the**
   A. prostate gland
   B. epididymis
   C. thyroid follicles
   D. pineal gland
   E. kidney tubules

57. **Which of the following statement is true for the thyroid gland?**
   A. The thyroid follicles are always lined by cuboidal epithelium irrespective of its state of activity
   B. The follicles are separated by sinusoids
   C. The parafollicular cells secrete parathormone
   D. The colloid is scanty when the gland is hyperactive
   E. The follicular cells secrete thyroxine and calcitonin

58. **The pars anterior of the hypophysis cerebri consists of**
   A. colloid filled follicles
   B. the chromophobes and the chromophils in almost equal proportion
   C. the chromophils arranged in the form of follicles
   D. the chromophobes which lie towards the periphery and the chromophils which lie towards the centre
   E. a network of nerve fibres and pituicytes

59. **Thyroid stimulating hormone is secreted by which cells of pituitary gland?**
   A. Acidophils
   B. Basophils
   C. Chromophobes
   D. Pituicytes

60. **Insulin is secreted by**
   A. acidophil cells of parathyroid
   B. beta cells of Islets of Langerhans
   C. chromophobes of pituitary
   D. parafollicular cells of thyroid

61. **The zona fasiculata of the suprarenal cortex**
   A. is the outermost layer
   B. is the thinnest of the three layers of the cortex
   C. is made up of cells which have vacuolated appearance in routine slides

Ans.   56. D   57. D   58. B   59. B   60. B

    D. is made up of cells arranged in one-cell thick columns

    E. secretes mineralocorticoids

62. The sensory ganglion can be distinguished from autonomic ganglion by all the following features *except* that the sensory neurons are

    A. larger in size

    B. pseudounipolar

    C. arranged singly

    D. surrounded by a well defined capsule of satellite cells

    E. having a nucleus which is usually central in position

63. All the following cells are present in the cerebral cortex *except*

    A. pyramidal cells

    B. stellate cells

    C. basket cells

    D. purkinje cells

    E. horizontal cells

64. Which of the following features differentiates the respiratory bronchiole from the terminal bronchiole?

    A. Absence of cartilage

    B. Absence of cilia

    C. Absence of glands

    D. Presence of alveoli on its wall

    E. Presence of goblet cells

65. In the larynx, stratified squamous epithelium is seen over

    A. vestibular folds

    B. vocal folds

    C. ventricle

    D. lower half of posterior surface of epiglottis

Directions: For each of the incomplete statements or questions below, one or more completions or answers is correct. Select

    A. if one 1,2 and 3 are correct;

    B. if only 1 and 3 are correct;

    C. if only 2 and 4 are correct;

    D. if only 4 is correct;

    E. if all are correct.

Ans.   61. C   62. C   63. D   64. D   65. B

66. **The cell membrane**
    1. is about 7.5 nm thick
    2. appears bilaminar under the electronmicroscope
    3. forms pinocytotic vesicles
    4. is freely permeable to all substances

67. **The rough endoplasmic reticulum**
    1. consists of flattened sacs or tubules
    2. has ribosomes attached on its internal surface
    3. is concerned primarily with the synthesis of proteins
    4. is also concerned with the synthesis of carbohydrates

68. **The mitochondria play an important role in**
    1. phagocytosis
    2. protein synthesis
    3. cell division
    4. energy production

69. **The pseudostratified epithelium**
    1. has nuclei in two or more layers
    2. has most of the cells resting on the basement membrane
    3. has some of the cells which do not reach the surface
    4. is only found in the respiratory passages

70. **The characters of collagen fibres are that they**
    1. run singly
    2. are inelastic
    3. contain flat nuclei
    4. form the ligaments and tendons

71. **The simple squamous epithelium lines the**
    1. blood vessels
    2. lymphatics
    3. alveoli
    4. ventricles of brain

72. **The brush border**
    1. consists of microvilli
    2. inhibits absorption
    3. is seen in cells lining the small intestine
    4. represents fine cilia

Ans.   66. B   67. B   68. D   69. B   70. C   71. A   72. B

73. **The reticuloendothelial system includes**
    1. histiocytes
    2. monocytes
    3. Kupffer cells
    4. plasma cells

74. **The articular cartilage**
    1. is a hyaline cartilage
    2. has a perichondrium on its surface
    3. receives nutrition from synovial fluid
    4. has numerous blood vessels

75. **The haversian systems**
    1. are present in compact and spongy bone
    2. once formed do not undergo remodelling
    3. are not connected with each other
    4. communicate with the medullary cavity and with the external surface through Volkman's canals

76. **The sinusoids**
    1. are wider than the capillaries
    2. have walls which may be incomplete at places
    3. also have macrophages in their walls
    4. connect capillaries with venules

77. **The B-lymphocytes**
    1. do not circulate through the thymus
    2. are responsible for graft rejection
    3. form plasma cells
    4. are not present in the blood

78. **The histological features of the lung include**
    1. a large number of alveoli lined by cuboidal epithelium
    2. bronchioles which are distinguished by the absence of cartilage in their walls
    3. connective tissue which is rich in collagen fibres
    4. extensive network of capillaries

79. **The esophagus**
    1. is lined by stratified squamous epithelium
    2. may have glands in the submucosa

Ans. 73. A 74. B 75. D 76. A 77. B 78. C

  3. has striated muscle in its upper two third part
  4. has no muscularis mucosae

80. The paneth cells are present in the
  1. appendix
  2. colon
  3. stomach
  4. small intestine

**81. The vermiform appendix can be distinguished by which of
the following features?**
  1. Narrow lumen
  2. Presence of only a few villi
  3. Abundant lymphoid tissue in the submucosa
  4. Numerous crypts in the lamina propria

**82. Which of the following statements are true regarding the
histological structure of the gall bladder?**
  1. Its mucous membrane is thrown into numerous folds
  2. Its mucous membrane is lined by simple columnar ciliated
      epithelium
  3. There are no goblet cells
  4. The muscularis mucosae is made up of outer longitudinal and
      inner circular muscle fibres

**83. Which of the following statements are true about the
structure of the liver?**
  1. The hepatocytes are arranged in the form of laminae each of
      which is two-cell thick
  2. The laminae are separated by the sinusoids
  3. Each hepatic lobule is supplied by one branch of hepatic
      artery
  4. Each portal lobule consists of parts of three hepatic lobules

84. The islets of Langerhans (in man)
  1. form endocrine part of the pancreas
  2. are restricted to the head of the pancreas
  3. have predominantly β-cells which secrete insulin
  4. have α-cells which tend to lie in the centre of the islet

---

Ans.   79. A   80. D   81. B   82. B   83. C   84. B

85. **Which of the following statements are true about the structure of the kidney?**
    1. The renal corpuscles are located in the cortex as well as the medulla
    2. The outer layer of the Bowman's capsule is lined by special cells called the podocytes
    3. The cells lining the distal convoluted tubules have numerous microvilli
    4. The cells of the proximal convoluted tubule are more eosinophillic than those of the distal convoluted tubule

86. **The juxtaglomerular apparatus**
    1. consists of modified smooth muscle cells of the afferent arteriole called macula densa
    2. consists of juxtaglomerular cells which are modified cells of distal convoluted tubule
    3. secretes an enzyme called renin produced by cells of the macula densa
    4. is concerned with the regulation of ion absorption by the renal tubule

87. **The features distinguishing the ductus deferens from the ureter are that the ductus deferens**
    1. has very thick muscle coat as compared to the size of the lumen
    2. has muscularis mucosae
    3. is lined by the pseudostratified columnar epithelium
    4. has mucous membrane which is thrown into circular folds

88. **The interstitial cells of testis**
    1. lie within the wall of the seminiferous tubule
    2. lie in the connective tissue that intervenes between the seminiferous tubules
    3. provide nutrition to the germ cells
    4. secrete testosterone

89. **A section through the epididymis shows**
    1. a mass of tubules cut up in various planes
    2. tubules lined by pseudostratified columnar epithelium
    3. tubules with a large well defined lumen
    4. corpora amylacea within the lumen of some of the tubules

---

Ans. 85. D 86. D 87. B 88. C 89. A

90. **Which of the following statements are true about the structure of the ovary?**
    1. It consists of a thin cortex and a thick medulla
    2. The cortex shows ovarian follicles at various stages of development
    3. Stroma has interstitial cells which secrete estrogen
    4. The medulla consists of numerous blood vessels

91. **A section through the fallopian tube shows**
    1. that mucous membrane is thrown into numerous branching folds
    2. that all the cells of the epithelium are ciliated
    3. an inner circular layer and an outer longitudinal layer of smooth muscle
    4. a few glands in the lamina propria

92. **The uterine endometrium consists of**
    1. a lining made up of pseudostratified columnar epithelium
    2. a stroma which is highly cellular
    3. branched tubular glands embedded in the stroma
    4. arteries of two types: straight and spiral

93. **The vagina has**
    1. a muscle coat made up of an outer layer of longitudinal and an inner layer of circular fibres
    2. submucosa with a few mucous glands
    3. mucosa lined by stratified squamous nonkeratinized epithelium
    4. lamina propria containing a few mucous glands

94. **The calcitonin producing cells**
    1. are scattered between the chief cells of the parathyroid gland
    2. belong to the APUD system
    3. lie just outside the basement membrane of the thyroid follicles
    4. are called parafollicular cells

95. **The APUD cell system**
    1. consists of endocrine cells
    2. is capable of taking up precursors of amines from the circulation
    3. form amines or peptides
    4. includes cells all of which show a positive chromaffin reaction

Ans.   90. C   91. B   92. C   93. B   94. C   95. A

96. **The various cells included in the APUD cell system are**
    1. the chief cells of the parathyroid
    2. chromophil cells of the adenohypophysis
    3. alpha cells of the pancreas
    4. cells of the adrenal medulla

97. **Which of the following statements are true about the retina?**
    1. Its outermost layer is made up of the rods and the cones
    2. The density of rods is greatest in the region around the macula lutea
    3. There are about 100 million cones in each retina
    4. The nuclei of rods and cones form the outer nuclear layer

98. **Which of the following statements are true for the cone cells of retina?**
    1. They are most numerous in the fovea centralis
    2. They are responsible for colour vision
    3. Their number is much less than that of rods
    4. They contain the pigment called visual purple

99. **The eyelid**
    1. is lined internally by conjunctiva which consists of stratified squamous epithelium resting on lamina propria
    2. has a tarsal plate made up of elastic cartilage
    3. externally is made up of skin which is usually devoid of sweat glands
    4. shows tarsal glands which are modified sebaceous glands

100. **The spiral organ of corti**
    1. is separated from the scala cochlae by the basilar membrane
    2. has three to four inner hair cells
    3. has a tunnel of corti enclosed by inner and outer rod cells
    4. has a single outer hair cell supported by Deiter's cells

Ans.   96. E   97. C   98. A   99. D   100. B

PART - III

GENETICS AND EMBRYOLOGY

CHAPTER 7

Genetics and Embryology

Directions: Each of the incomplete statements or questions below is followed by four or five suggested completions or answers. Select the one which is BEST in each case.

1. **Somatic cell is male has**
   A. 22 pairs of autosomes and two X chromosomes
   B. 22 pairs of autosomes and two Y chromosomes
   C. 22 pairs of autosomes and a pair each of X and Y chromosomes
   D. 22 pairs of autosomes and one X and one Y chromosomes

2. **In a DNA molecule adenine always forms a linkage with**
   A. guanine   B. cytosine
   C. thymine   D. uracil

3. **The part of a DNA molecule bearing the code for a complete polypeptide chain is called a**
   A. cistron   B. chalone
   C. codon   D. anticondon
   E. operon

4. **Which of the following is *not* a character of dominant inheritance?**
   A. Every diseased person has a parent who manifests the disease
   B. The disease appears in every generation
   C. Unaffected persons can transmit the disease
   D. The chances of the children being normal or diseased are equal if one of the parents is diseased and the other is a normal individual

Ans. 1. D   2. C   3. A   4. C

5. The term embryo is used for the developing individual during the first
   A. two weeks
   B. four weeks
   C. six weeks
   D. eight weeks
   E. ten weeks

6. Sex of a baby is determined at the time
   A. of gametogenesis
   B. of fertilization
   C. when gonads start developing
   D. when the gonads become active to secrete sex hormones
   E. when the hypophysis cerebri becomes active to secrete gonadotrophins

7. From the time of birth upto puberty the number of oogonia
   A. increase tremendously
   B. increase slightly
   C. remains constant
   D. decreases

8. In relation to the developing Graafian follicle
   A. a number of follicles start developing in one ovarian cycle
   B. the granulosa cells form the theca interna
   C. the cells of theca interna develop into luteal cells
   D. the ovum is surrounded by corona radiata in the follicle
   E. unruptured follicles give rise to corpora lutea

9. Ovulation
   A. occurs 14 days after the onset of the menstrual cycle
   B. occurs 14 days before the onset of the next menstrual cycle
   C. always occurs in the middle of the menstrual cycle irrespective of the length of the cycle
   D. can occur at any time during the menstrual cycle

10. The average life of the ovum after ovulation is about
    A. 8 hours
    B. 24 hours
    C. 3 days
    D. 5 days
    E. 7 days

Ans.   5. D   6. B   7. D   8. A   9. B   10. B

11. **The fertilization of ovum usually occurs in the**
    A. peritoneal cavity
    B. fallopian tube
    C. body of uterus
    D. cervix uteri
    E. vagina

12. **The fertilized ovum starts inplantation usually on the**
    A. 1st day
    B. 3rd day
    C. 7th day
    D. 15th day
    E. 20th day

13. **Which of the following statement is *not* true about oogenesis?**
    A. The number of germ cells does not increase after birth
    B. The secondary oocyte has only 23 chromosomes
    C. One primary oocyte give rise to only one ovum
    D. During the ovarian cycle usually only one follicle reaches maturity
    E. The second meiotic division is completed before fertilization

14. **The corpus luteum of pregnancy is active for**
    A. 14 days
    B. 1-2 months
    C. 2-3 months
    D. 3-4 months
    E. throughout pregnancy

15. **The cells surrounding the oocyte in a mature Graafian follicle are called**
    A. granulosa cells
    B. cumulus oophori .'s
    C. corona radiata
    D. discus proligerus
    E. theca interna

16. **In relation to the mature spermatozoon**
    A. the head is completely covered by the acrosomic cap
    B. the mitochondrial sheath surrounds the middle and principal pieces

Ans.   11. B   12. C   13. E   14. D   15. B

C. the principal piece consists of a pair of central tubules surrounded by nine pairs of tubules only

D. the acrosomic cap is the most likely source of hyaluronidase which is essential for fertilization of ovum

E. is capable of fertilising the ovum when it leaves the testis

17. **The secretory phase of uterine cycle is characterised by**
   A. endometrium which is about 5-7 mm thick
   B. uterine glands which show saw-toothed appearance
   C. growth of spiral arteries
   D. endometrium divisible into three strata
   E. all the above features

18. **The cyclical changes occur in the**
   A. entire uterus
   B. only the body of the uterus
   C. body of the uterus and the isthmus part of the cervix
   D. only in the cervix uteri
   E. only in the fundus

19. **The most important event resulting in implantation of the fertilized ovum is the**
   A. cleavage
   B. separation of trophoblast cells and the inner cell mass
   C. formation of blastocyst
   D. disintegration of zona pellucida
   E. formation of decidua

20. **The intraembryonic mesoderm is mainly derived from the**
   A. notochord
   B. primitive streak
   C. trophoblasts
   D. prochordal plate

21. **The fate of the notochord is that it**
   A. disappear completely
   B. persists as the vertebral column
   C. persists as the nucleus pulposus
   D. forms spinal cord
   E. none of the above

Ans. 16. D 17. E 18. C 19. D 20. B 21. C

22. **The prochordal plate**
    A. lies near the caudal end of the embryonic disc
    B. is the future buccopharyngeal membrane
    C. is trilaminar in structure
    D. lies cranial to the septum transversum before the formation of head fold
    E. closes the distal end of the hind gut

23. **Which of the following is *not* a function of the placenta?**
    A. Exchange of CO_2 and O_2
    B. Exchange of nutrition
    C. Secretion of hormones
    D. Formation of blood
    E. Prevention of antigen-antibody reaction between maternal and foetal blood

24. **The usual amount of amniotic fluid at full term is**
    A. 100 cc
    B. 500 cc
    C. 1000 cc
    D. 2000 cc
    E. 3000 cc

25. **Placenta praevia is a condition in which**
    A. the umbilical cord is attached near the margin of placenta
    B. there is an additional lobe of placenta
    C. the placenta is attached in the lower half of the body of the uterus
    D. the placenta is thin and membranous

26. **The amniotic fluid**
    A. allows mobility of foetus
    B. protects the foetus from external injury
    C. helps in parturition
    D. provides support for the foetus
    E. has all the above functions

27. **Which of the following statements is true about the development of vertebral column?**
    A. It is formed from the lateral part of somites
    B. Each vertebra is formed from two adjacent sclerotomes

Ans.   22. B   23. D   24. C   25. C   26. E

    C. The transverse processes are segmental in origin

    D. The remnants of notochord are present in the body of the vertebra

    E. Failure of fusion of the two halves of the neural arch results in hemivertebra

28. **Which of the following epithelia is derived from the mesoderm?**
    A. Inner lining of eyelid
    B. Endothelium of blood vessels
    C. Lining of biliary passages
    D. Lining of most of the urinary bladder
    E. All the above

29. **Which of the following epithelia is *not* a derivative of endoderm?**
    A. Lining of the larynx
    B. Lining epithelium of pancreatic ducts
    C. Lining of the lower part of rectum
    D. Lining of the trigone of urinary bladder
    E. Epithelium of tongue

30. **Which of the following is *not* a derivative of mesenchymal cells?**
    A. Haemocytoblast
    B. Mast cell
    C. Myoblast
    D. Osteoblast
    E. Neuroblast

31. **Which of the following muscles is not developed from mesoderm?**
    A. Arrectores pilorum
    B. Ciliary muscle
    C. Muscles of the iris
    D. Muscles of the tongue
    E. Stapedius

32. **Which is the most precarious period of prenatal development?**
    A. Conception to 2 month

Ans.   27. B   28. B   29. D   30. E   31. C

B. 2nd to 4th month
C. 4th to 6th month
D. Third trimester

33. Oogenesis gets arrested at the state of
A. prophase I
B. prophase II
C. diakinesis
D. anaphase I

34. All the following structures are mesodermal in origin *except*
A. serous membranes
B. lymphoid tissue
C. brain
D. heart

35. Inner lining of which of the following structures is endodermal in origin?
A. Aorta
B. Ureter
C. Nasal cavity
D. Trachea

36. All the following are derivatives of endoderm *except*
A. pituitary gland
B. pancreas
C. parathyroid gland
D. thyroid gland

37. Which of the following features pertain to inborn errors of metabolism?
A. Sex-linked disease
B. Most often inherited as an autosomal dominant
C. Expressed only in homozygotes
D. Prenatal diagnosis possible by ultrasound examination

38. Which of the following is *not* a function of placenta?
A. Removal of excretory products
B. Prevent mixing of maternal and fetal blood
C. Complete protection from viruses
D. Produce progesteron

Ans.   32. A   33. A   34. C   35. D   36. A   37. C   38. C

39. **In third degree placenta praevia placenta is attached in such a way that**
    A. its edge just extends into the lower uterine segment
    B. its edge covers the closed internal os but not the dilated os
    C. it covers the internal os even when it is fully dilated
    D. its edge extends upto the internal os but does not cover it at all

40. **A painless midline swelling just below hyoid bone could be due to which of the following conditions?**
    A. Thyroglossal cyst
    B. Branchial cyst
    C. Undescended thymus
    D. Ectopic parathyroid gland

41. **Which of the following is the commonest congenital anomaly of face or palate?**
    A. Unilateral cleft palate
    B. Median cleft lip
    C. Unilateral cleft lip
    D. Cleft lip with cleft palate

42. **Lingual tonsil shows all the following features *except***
    A. it may be present under the mucosa of tongue
    B. it may be present embedded within the muscle tissue of tongue
    C. it may be located under the tongue
    D. it produces difficulty in swallowing

43. **Which of the following developmental patterns is common to sweat glands, mammary glands, lacrimal gland and prostate glands?**
    A. All develop from ectoderm
    B. All develop under the influence of pituitary hormone
    C. All develop by invagination of epithelium into underlying mesenchyme
    D. All atrophy with age

44. **Which of the following is a derivative of the first pharyngeal pouch?**
    A. Tonsil
    B. Thymus
    C. Pharyngotympanic tube

Ans.   39. B   40. A   41. C   42. C   43. C

D. Superior parathyroid
E. Inferior parathyroid

45. Which of the following muscles is *not* a derivative of the second branchial arch?
A. Buccinator
B. Stapedius
C. Platysma
D. Anterior belly of digastric
E. Orbicularis oculi

46. Which of the following is *not* a derivative of the first branchial arch?
A. Incus
B. Sphenomandibular ligament
C. Mandible
D. Levator palati
E. Anterior belly of digastric muscle

47. Which of the following structures does *not* contribute to the development of tongue?
A. Tuberculum impar
B. Lingual swellings
C. Caudal part of hypobranchial eminence
D. Occipital myotomes

48. The first permanent tooth to erupt is
A. central incisor
B. lateral incisor
C. canine
D. first premolar
E. first molar

49. Which of the following bones is completely formed in membrane?
A. Frontal
B. Occipital
C. Inferior nasal concha
D. Ethmoid
E. Mandible

Ans.   44. C   45. D   46. D   47. C   48. E   49. A

50. **Adjoining digits are fused in**
    A. brachydactyly
    B. synphalangia
    C. arachnodactyly
    D. syndactyly
    E. syndesmosis

51. **All the following structures are derivatives of the midgut *except* the**
    A. jejunum
    B. caecum
    C. ascending colon
    D. descending colon
    E. appendix

52. **The main pancreatic duct represents**
    A. the duct of the ventral pancreatic bud only
    B. the duct of the dorsal pancreatic bud only
    C. the duct of the ventral pancreatic bud proximally and the duct of the dorsal pancreatic bud distally
    D. the ducts of the ventral pancreatic bud, the dorsal pancreatic bud and the hepatic bud

53. **Which part of the G.I.T. develops from the part of primitive gut in the region of attachment of vitellointestinal duct?**
    A. Rectum
    B. Caecum
    C. Appendix
    D. Ileum

54. **Dudenum does not form part of physiological hernia during intrauterine life because**
    A. It has no dorsal mesogastrium
    B. Cystic bud arises from it
    C. It is attached to posterior abdominal wall by ligament of Treitz
    D. It is derived from foregut and midgut

55. **During development the midgut loop undergoes anticlockwise rotation through**
    A. 90°
    B. 180°

Ans. 50. D 51. D 52. C 53. D 54. C

C. 270°
D. 360°

56. All the following statements are true for **tracheo-esophageal fistula** *except* that it is
A. a common neonatal emergency
B. due to defective development of tracheoesophageal septum
C. usually associated with atresia of esophagus
D. generally associated with oligamnios

57. **Rectovesical fistula** occurs due to defective development of
A. cloacal membrane
B. urorectal septum
C. allantois
D. absorption of mesonephric ducts

58. Which of the following is *not* derived from **foregut endothelium?**
A. Kupffer cells
B. Hepatocytes
C. Beta cells of pancreas
D. Lining of biliary tract

59. **Accessory pancreatic duct** develops from
A. Dorsal pancreatic bud
B. Ventral pancreatic bud
C. Both dorsal and ventral pancreatic buds
D. Endoderm of midgut

60. Which part of the gut temporarily lies outside the abdominal cavity in the extraembryonic coelom?
A. Foregut
B. Duodenal loop
C. Midgut
D. Hindgut

61. **Exomphalos** is a condition related to
A. defective development of urinary bladder
B. non-return of midgut loop into the abdominal cavity
C. defective development of heart
D. abnormal protrusion of the eyeball
E. defective development of the phallus

Ans.   55. C   56. D   57. B   58. A   59. A   60. C   61. B

\

62. **Just after the midgut loop returns to the abdominal cavity the caecum lies**
    A. just below the liver
    B. under the spleen
    C. in the left iliac fossa
    D. in the right iliac fossa

63. **Which of the following statements is true about the development of spleen?**
    A. It develops in the ventral mesogastrium
    B. It develops from the mesenchymal cells
    C. It develops from the endoderm of foregut
    D. It develops from coelomic epithelium on the posterior abdominal wall close to the left kidney

64. **The fate of the left horn of the sinus venosus is that it**
    A. disappears completely
    B. is absorbed into the right atrium
    C. is absorbed into the left atrium
    D. forms the whole of the coronary sinus
    E. forms only the medial part of the coronary sinus

65. **What is the fate of the bulbus cordis (the conus)?**
    A. Gets incorporated into the right ventricle
    B. Gets incorporated into the left ventricle
    C. Gets incorporated into both the ventricles
    D. Gives rise to the pulmonary trunk and the aorta
    E. Gets incorporated into the two atria

66. **Ductus arteriosus**
    A. connects pulmonary vein to dorsal aorta
    B. functional closure occurs after one week of birth
    C. complete obliteration results in formation of ligamentum teres
    D. develops from left sixth arch artery

67. **Which of the following vessels will contain the highest oxygen content during intrauterine life?**
    A. Ascending aorta
    B. Ductus arteriosus
    C. Ductus venosus
    D. Umbilical vein

Ans. 62. A 63. B 64. E 65. C 66. D 67. D

68. **Which statement is true about development of heart?**
  A. Common atrial chamber is the most cranial part of fused heart tube
  B. Heart tubes fuse from caudal to cranial side
  C. Bulbus cordis gets incorporated into common atrial chamber
  D. Heart tube invaginates the pericardial cavity from dorsal side.

69. **Each horn of the sinus venosus receives the following vessels** *except*
  A. vitelline vein
  B. umbilical vein
  C. common cardinal vein
  D. subcardinal vein

70. **Defective development of septum of His can lead to of the following defects** *except*
  A. ostium primum defect
  B. interventricular septal defect
  C. persistent atrioventricular canal
  D. transposition of great vessels

71. **Which of the following components does** *not* **contribute to the formation of the inferior vena cava?**
  A. The right supracardinal vein
  B. The right subcardinal vein
  C. The right supracardinal-subcardinal anastomosis
  D. The terminal part of the right posterior cardinal vein
  E. The right hepatocardiac channel

72. **The right fourth aortic arch**
  A. disappears completely
  B. forms part of the right common carotid artery
  C. forms part of the right subclavian artery
  D. forms the brachiocephalic trunk
  E. forms the right internal carotid artery

73. **Which of the following parts of the renal tubule is developed from the ureteric bud?**
  A. Bowman's capsule
  B. Convoluted tubules
  C. Loop of Henle

Ans.   68. D   69. D   70. D   71. D   72. C

    D. Collecting ducts

    E. All the above

74. **In non-rotation of the kidney, the hilum is directed**
    A. anteromedially
    B. anteriorly
    C. posteriorly
    D. laterally
    E. medially

75. **The epithelium of most of the urinary bladder is derived from**
    A. definitive urogenital sinus
    B. primitive urogenital sinus
    C. cloaca
    D. vesicourethral canal
    E. mesonephric duct

76. **The primordial germ cells are derived from the**
    A. allantois
    B. yolk sac endoderm
    C. coelomic epithelium
    D. mesonephros
    E. mesenchyme of genital ridge

77. **Which of the following is a remnant of the paramesonephric duct in male?**
    A. Appendix of epididymis
    B. Appendix of testis
    C. Paradidymis
    D. Superior aberrant ductules
    E. Inferior aberrant ductules

78. **All the following are the derivatives of the neural crest *except* the**
    A. neurons of sympathetic ganglia
    B. neurons of geniculate ganglion
    C. Schwann cells
    D. oligodendrocytes
    E. melanoblasts of the skin

79. **The cerebellum develops from the**
    A. alar laminae of the myelencephalon

Ans.   73. D   74. B   75. D   76. B   77. B   78. D

    B. basal laminae of the myelencephalon
    C. alar laminae of the metencephalon
    D. basal laminae of the metencephalon
    E. alar laminae of the myelencephalon and the metencephalon

80. Efferent cranial nerves develop from neurones in
    A. alar lamina
    B. basal lamina
    C. roof plate
    D. floor plate

81. Cerebellum develops from
    A. diencephalon
    B. mesencephalon
    C. metencephalon
    D. myelencephalon

82. All the features are true for ductus venosus *except*
    A. it connects portal vein with inferior vena cava
    B. oxygenated blood by passes the liver through it
    C. obliteration after birth forms ligamentum venosum
    D. it develops from supracardinal vein

83. Which of the following statements regarding ectopia vesicae is true?
    A. The anterior wall of urinary bladder is exposed on the surface
    B. Infraumbilical part of anterior abdominal wall is not developed
    C. Often associated with hypospadias
    D. Person can lead a normal life

84. All the following are features of Anencephalic baby *except*
    A. primary defect is failure of closure of cranial part of neural tube
    B. cranial vault is missing
    C. bulging forehead
    D. bulging eyes

85. All the following statements pertain to spina bifida occulta *except*
    A. there is defective development of spinal cord
    B. there is defective fusion of vertebral arches

Ans.   79. C   80. A   81. C   82. D   83. B   84. C

C. there is no associated neural deficit

D. there is no associated defect in meninges

Directions: For each of the incomplete statements or questions below, one or more completions or answers is correct. Select

A. if only 1,2 and 3 are correct;

B. if only 1 and 3 are correct;

C. if only 2 and 4 are correct;

D. if only 4 is correct;

E. if all are correct.

---

86. **Which of the following is/are true for Trisomy?**
    1. It is characterised by the presence of 69 chromosomes
    2. Occurs due to the fusion of a diploid and a haploid gamete
    3. Trisomy of X chromosome occurs in Turner's syndrome
    4. Trisomy of chromosome 21 results in Mongolism

87. **Which of the following statements are true about mutations?**
    1. Mutations can occur only in germ cells
    2. The mutant gene is transmitted to future generations just like the original gene
    3. The mutation rate decreases with increasing age of the individuals
    4. The mutation rate increases with exposure of germ cells to high temperature

88. **Which of the following structures normally contribute to the formation of the placenta?**
    1. Decidua capsularis
    2. Decidua basalis
    3. Splanchnopleuric extraembryonic mesoderm
    4. Trophoblast

89. **The placental membrane in the human placenta consists of**
    1. endothelium of foetal capillaries
    2. cytotrophoblast
    3. syncytiotrophoblast
    4. maternal capillary endothelium

90. **Which of the following statements are true about the placenta?**
    1. It does not allow the passage of any harmful organism

Ans. 85. A   86. D   87.   88. C   89. A

2. Its maternal surface is smooth
3. The placental membrane becomes thinner as the pregnancy advances due to the disappearance of syncytiotrophoblasts
4. Usually the placenta is formed in the upper uterine segment

91. Which of the following bones are partly formed in cartilage and partly in membrane?
1. Mandible
2. Occipital
3. Sphenoid
4. Frontal

92. Which of the following statements are true about the metaphysis?
1. It develops from secondary ossification centre
2. It is the site of minimum calcium turnover
3. It is not very vascular
4. It is frequently the site of infection

93. Which of the following statements are true about the development of bone?
1. All bone is of mesodermal origin
2. Osteoclasts play no role in the development of bone
3. The bones grow by appositional growth
4. The increase in length of the bone takes place mainly by the growth of the epiphysis

94. Which of the following statements are true about the development of skin?
1. The epidermis is derived from the dermatome of the somites
2. The sweat glands are ectodermal in origin
3. The melanoblasts of the epidermis are derived from the mesenchymal cells
4. The dermis is mesodermal in origin

95. Which of the following skeletal elements are derivatives of the third pharyngeal arch?
1. Greater cornu of hyoid bone
2. Upper part of body of hyoid bone
3. Lower part of body of hyoid bone
4. Thyroid cartilage

Ans.   90. D   91. A   92. D   93. B   94. C   95. B

96. The hypobranchial eminence contributes to the development of
    1. anterior two third of the tongue
    2. posterior one third of the tongue
    3. thyroid cartilage
    4. epiglottis

97. The upper lip is derived from the
    1. maxillary processes
    2. frontonasal process
    3. mesoderm of the second pharyngeal arch
    4. mesoderm of the first pharyngeal arch

98. Which of the following statements are true about the development of palate?
    1. The premaxilla (which carries the incisor teeth) is derived from the maxillary process
    2. The frontonasal process froms the major part of palate
    3. Non-fusion of the palatal process with the frontonasal process results in a median cleft palate
    4. The fusion of palatal processes begins anteriorly and proceeds backwards

99. Which of the following are derivatives of frontonasal process?
    1. Lateral wall of nasal cavity
    2. Medial wall of nasal cavity
    3. Muscles of the upper tip
    4. Median part of the upper tip

100. Which of the following are derivatives of the maxillary process?
    1. Upper part of cheek
    2. Floor of nasal cavity
    3. Lower eyelid
    4. Upper eyelid

101. Which of the following contribute to the formation of the lesser sac?
    1. Left pneumatoenteric recess
    2. Elongation and folding of the greater omentum

Ans.   96. C   97. A   98. D   99. C   100. A

3. Cranial extension of the left pneumatoenteric recess
4. Rotation of stomach

102. Which of the following statements are true about rotation of gut?
1. The duodenal loop herniates out in the extraembryonic coelom and undergoes rotation
2. Viewed from the ventral side the rotation is clockwise
3. The post arterial segment returns to the abdominal cavity before the pre-arterial segment
4. In reversed rotation the transverse colon crosses behind the superior mesenteric artery

103. The duodenum develops from
1. foregut endothelium
2. midgut endothelium
3. splanchnopleuric mesoderm
4. somatopleuric mesoderm

104. The derivatives of the hindgut include
1. sigmoid colon
2. urinary bladder
3. rectum
4. urethra

105. The cloaca communicates with the
1. hindgut
2. paramesonephric duct
3. allantois
4. amniotic cavity

106. The liver is developed from the
1. septum transversum
2. vitelline veins
3. umbilical veins
4. hepatic bud

107. The derivatives of the dorsal mesogastrium include
1. gastrosplenic ligament
2. lienorenal ligament
3. gastrophrenic ligament
4. gastrohepatic ligament

Ans.   101. E 102. D 103. A 104. E 105. B 106. E 107. A

108. Which of the following statements are true about the development of the diaphragm?
1. It starts developing in the neck and later migrates to its definitive position
2. Septum transversum forms the central tendon
3. Mesoderm of the body wall forms its peripheral portion
4. Pleuroperitoneal membranes form the anterolateral parts of the diaphragm

109. The interatrial septum is formed by
1. spiral septum
2. septum secondum
3. septum spurium
4. septum primum

110. The features of Fallot's tetrology include
1. interatrial septal defect
2. interventricular septal defect
3. aortic stenosis
4. pulmonary stenosis

111. The fate of sinus venosus is that its
1. right horn is absorbed into the right atrium
2. left horn is absorbed into the left atrium
3. left horn forms part of the coronary sinus
4. right horn forms part of the superior vena cava

112. The ventricles are derived from
1. the primitive ventricular chamber
2. the atrioventricular canals
3. the proximal part of the bulbus cordis
4. the distal part of the bulbus cordis

113. The fate of left sixth arch artery is that it
1. disappears completely
2. forms left common carotid
3. forms part of arch of aorta
4. forms ductus arteriosus

114. The changes which occur in the foetal circulation at birth include
1. closure of foramen ovale

Ans.   108. A 109. C 110. C 111. B 112. A 113. D

2. decrease in pressure in right atrium
3. contraction of umbilical arteries
4. formation of pulmonary arteries

115. The superior vena cava is derived from the right
1. anterior cardinal vein
2. posterior cardinal vein
3. common cardinal vein
4. right horn of sinus venosus

116. The arch of aorta is derived from the
1. left horn of the aortic sac
2. left fourth aortic arch
3. ventral part of the aortic sac
4. dorsal part of the aortic sac

117. Which of the following statements are true about the neural tube?
1. It develops from the ectoderm overlying the notochordal process
2. The special visceral neurons are located nearest to the sulcus limitans
3. The alar laminae contain sensory neurons
4. The myelencephalon forms the medulla oblongata and the cerebellum

118. The bulbopontine extension gives rise to the
1. pontine nuclei
2. cerebellar nuclei
3. olivary nucleus.   '
4. nuclei of reticular formation in medulla and pons

119. The hypophysis cerebri develops form
1. ectodermal Rathke's pouch which arises just caudal to the buccopharyngeal membrane
2. ectodermal Rathke's pouch which arises just cranial to the buccopharyngeal membrane
3. a down growth from the floor of the telencehephalon
4. a downgrowth from the floor of the diencephalon

Ans.   114. A   115. B   116. A   117. B   118. B   119. C

120. **Which of the following are derivatives of mesonephric duct?**
    1. Ureteric bud
    2. Urethra caudal to the opening of ejaculatory ducts
    3. Vas deferens
    4. Seminiferous tubules

121. **Which of the following are derivatives of the para-mesonephric duct?**
    1. Fallopian tube
    2. Body of uterus
    3. Cervix uteri
    4. Gartner's duct

122. **The prostatic part of the urethra is derived from the**
    1. vesicourethral canal
    2. phallic part of urogenital sinus
    3. pelvic part of urogenital sinus
    4. mesonephric tubule

123. **Which of the following statements is/are true about the development of kidney?**
    1. It develops in the lumbar region
    2. It is partly mesodermal and partly endodermal in origin
    3. The uretheric bud forms the collecting ducts and the distal convoluted tubules
    4. The metanephric cap forms the secretory part of the renal tubule

124. **The mesonephric tubules in the male**
    1. form efferent ductules of the testis
    2. form superior aberrant ductules
    3. form inferior aberrant ductules
    4. disappear completely

125. **The mesonephric tubules in the female form**
    1. epoophoron
    2. Gartner's duct
    3. paraoophoron
    4. fallopian tube

Ans.   120. B   121. A   122. B   123. D   124. A   125. B

Directions: Each question consists of an assertion and a reason. Answers should be choosen as follows:

    A. if the assertion and reason are true statements and the reason is a correct explanation of the assertion;

    B. if the assertion and reason are true statements but the reason is not a correct explanation of the assertion;

    C. if the assertion is true but the reason is a false statement;

    D. if the assertion is false but the reason is a true statement;

    E. if both assertion and reason are false statements.

126. **Monozygotic twins always have the same sex**
Because
they always lie in the same chorionic sac

127. **Haemophilia is never transmitted from father to son**
Because
the disease is linked with X chromosome

128. **The sperms taken from the testis are capable of fertilizing the ovum**
Because
they are fully motile

129. **The entire preovulatory period of the menstrual cycle is regarded as the 'safe period' as far as prevention of pregnancy is concerned**
Because
the endometrium is not in the secretory phase during this period

130. **Non-fusion of the maxillary process with the lateral nasal process results in unilateral hare lip**
Because
the upper lip is derived from these two processes

131. **Spina bifida occulta is incompatible with postnatal life**
Because
it this region the spinal cord lies exposed on the surface

132. **In a woman having 34 days menstrual cycle the ovulation will occur on the 17th day**
Because
ovulation takes place in the middle of the cycle

Ans.   126. C 127. A 128. E 129. D 130. E 131. E 132. E

133. **The position of the superior parathyroid is more variable**
Because
its development is closely related to the development of thymus

134. **Sometimes the inferior vena cava crosses anterior to the right ureter**
Because
the ureteric bud grows posterior to the developing inferior vena cava

135. **In hypospadias the urethra opens somewhere on the undersurface of the penis**
Because
the urethral folds fuse only partially

136. **Immediately after birth the pressure in the right ventricle increases**
Because
the lungs expand and blood starts circulating through them

137. **The big toe develops on the postaxial border but comes to lie on the medial side**
Because
the lower limb undergoes adduction and medial rotation during development

138. **Failure of union between the derivatives of metanephrogenic cap and the ureteric bud leads to polycystic kidney**
Because
the urine accumulates in the proximal tubules and cannot pass into collecting tubules

139. **Cryptorchidism may lead to sterility**
Because
the external genital organs are not developed properly

140. **Oligohydramnios is usually associated with multiple deformities of the foetus**
Because
there is direct pressure of uterine walls on the skull, limbs and trunk

---

Ans.   133. E   134. C   135. A   136. D   137. D   138. A   139. C   140. A

PART- IV

NEUROANATOMY

CHAPTER 8

Neuroanatomy

Directions: Each of the incomplete statements or questions below is followed by four or five suggested completions or answers. Select the one which is BEST in each case.

1. **The cerebrospinal fluid**
   A. formed by arachnoid villi
   B. absorbed by ependyma
   C. present in the subarachnoid space
   D. composition is similar to that of plasma
   E. enters the subarachnoid space through foramen of Monro

2. **Which of the following statements is true for the cranial dura mater?**
   A. It is made up of a single layer
   B. It contains venous sinuses
   C. It is separated from arachnoid mater by cerebrospinal fluid
   D. It is insensitive to pain
   E. It gives extensions along all the cranial nerves

3. **Which of the following statements is *not* true for the spinal dura mater?**
   A. It is equivalent to the meningeal layer of cranial dura mater
   B. External vertebral venous plexus lies between it and the periosteum of vertebral canal
   C. It terminates at the level of the second sacral vertebra
   D. It extends into the intervertebral foramina and fuses with the periosteum of the vertebrae
   E. It terminates caudally as the filum terminale

Ans.   1. C   2. B   3. E

4. **The pia mater**
   A. is an avascular membrane
   B. loosely invests the brain and spinal cord
   C. is sensitive to pain
   D. forms two ligamenta denticulata which help in fixing the spinal cord
   E. extends beyond the conus medullaris as coccygeal ligament

5. **The arachnoid mater**
   A. is a vascular membrane
   B. extends upto the second sacral vertebra
   C. gives extensions to all the cranial nerves
   D. dips into sulci and fissures of brain and spinal cord
   E. is not connected to the pia mater

6. **The bipolar neurons are present in the**
   A. dorsal root ganglion
   B. sympathetic ganglion
   C. cochlear ganglion
   D. trigeminal ganglion
   E. mesencephalic nucleus

7. **The cells which provide myelin sheath in the central nervous system are the**
   A. astrocytes   B. oligodendrocytes
   C. microglia   D. Schwann cells
   E. internuncial neurons

8. **The regenerating axons grow at an average rate of**
   A. 0.1 mm/day   B. 1.0 mm./day
   C. 5.0 mm/day   D. 1.0 cm/day

9. **The spinal cord**
   A. extends from the upper border of atlas to the second sacral vertebra
   B. is broadest at the level of lumbar enlargement
   C. shows a deep fissure on its dorsal aspect
   D. has a lower tapering end called conus medullaris
   E. has 33 segments

Ans.   4. D   5. B   6. C   7. B   8. B   9. D

10. **Which of the following statements is *not* true regarding the blood supply of spinal cord?**
    A. It is supplied by anterior and posterior spinal branches of vertebral artery
    B. The two posterior spinal arteries supply two thirds of the cross sectional area of spinal cord
    C. Radicular arteries reinforce anterior and posterior spinal arteries
    D. Arteria radicularis magna usually arises from one of the segmental arteries in lower thoracic or upper lumbar vertebral levels
    E. Venous drainage is into segmental veins

11. **At birth the lower end of the spinal cord usually lies at the level of**
    A. lower border of L1 vertebra
    B. lower border of L3 vertebra
    C. lower border of L5 vertebra
    D. lower border of S2 vertebra
    E. lower border of S5 vertebra

12. **Which of the following statements is *not* true for spinal nerves?**
    A. There are 31 pairs of spinal nerves
    B. The dorsal ramus is purely sensory
    C. The ventral root is purely motor
    D. The dorsal rami do not form plexuses
    E. The ventral roots also contain preganglionic autonomic fibres

13. **The sensation of touch is carried by**
    A. anterior spinothalamic tract only
    B. lateral spinothalamic tract only
    C. anterior spinothalamic and posterior column tracts
    D. lateral spinothalamic and posterior column tracts
    E. posterior column tracts only

14. **Which of the following statements is true for the posterior spinocerebellar tract?**
    A. It lies in the posterior funiculus
    B. Most of its fibres arise from the ipsilateral dorsal nucleus of spinal cord

---

Ans.   10. B   11. B   12. B   13. C   14. B

C. It reaches the cerebellum through superior cerebellar peduncle
D. It carries proprioceptive impulses from upper limbs
E. It terminates mainly in the neocerebellum

15. **The posterior column tracts carry all the following sensations** *except*
    A. tactile localisation
    B. proprioceptive from skeletal muscle, joints and tendons
    C. sensation of bladder distension
    D. pain
    E. stereognosis

16. **Which of the following statements is true for pyramidal tracts?**
    A. All the fibres arise from motor cortex
    B. They pass through the posterior limb of internal capsule
    C. They pass through the medial two thirds of the crus cerebri
    D. Majority of their fibres cross rostral to the sensory decussation in medulla oblongata
    E. Injury to these tracts at the level of midbrain results in contralateral paresis and hypotonia of muscles

17. **The medulla oblongata**
    A. lies behind dorsum sellae
    B. is demarcated from the lower border of pons by a groove in which VI, VII, VIII and IX nerves are attached
    C. shows gracile and cuneate tubercles on its ventral aspect
    D. is connected to the cerebellum by the inferior cerebellar peduncles
    E. gives attachment to the hypoglossal nerve along anterolateral sulcus

18. **Which of the following cranial nerve nuclei does** *not* **lie in the medulla oblongata?** -
    A. Dorsal nucleus of vagus
    B. Nucleus of tractus solitarius
    C. Spinal nucleus of trigeminal nerve
    D. Nucleus of facial nerve
    E. Ventral cochlear nucleus

Ans. 15. D   16. B   17. D   18. D

19. **Which of the following arteries does *not* supply medulla oblongata?**
    A. Anterior spinal artery
    B. Posterior spinal artery
    C. Anterior inferior cerebellar artery
    D. Posterior inferior cerebellar artery
    E. Direct branches from vertebral artery

20. **The fourth ventricle**
    A. communicates with the third ventricle through foramen of Monro
    B. shows facial colliculus formed by the underlying nucleus of facial nerve
    C. roof in its upper part is formed by the superior medullary velum and superior cerebellar peduncles
    D. has only three recesses
    E. has a median aperture in the upper part of its roof

21. **The pons**
    A. shows a groove on its ventral surface, in which lies the basilar venous plexus
    B. forms floor of the upper part of the IV ventricle
    C. has no nucleus belonging to the somatic efferent group
    D. is connected to the cerebellum by superior cerebellar peduncles
    E. gives attachment to the fourth and fifth cranial nerves

22. **The trapezoid body in formed by the crossing axons of**
    A. cochlear nuclei
    B. superior olivary nuclei
    C. nucleus of trapezoid body
    D. all the above nuclei

23. **The medial lemniscus in the pons**
    A. forms a transverse band close to the midline
    B. lies lateral to the lateral spinothalamic tract
    C. consists of third order neurons
    D. forms part of hearing pathway
    E. terminates in the ventroposterior medial nucleus of thalamus

Ans. 19. C   20. C   21. B   22. D   23. A

24. **The midbrain**
    A. passes through the tentorial notch
    B. shows four colliculi on its ventral aspect
    C. forms uppermost part of the floor of IV ventricle
    D. forms anterolateral boundary of interpeduncular fossa
    E. has none of the above properties

25. **The midbrain at the level of inferior colliculus shows**
    A. red nucleus
    B. mesencephalic nucleus
    C. Edinger-Westphal nucleus
    D. pretectal nucleus
    E. none of the above

26. **The thalamus**
    A. has a superior surface which is completely covered by ependyma
    B. forms the anterior boundary of interventricular foramen
    C. can be seen on the base of brain
    D. is related laterally to internal capsule
    E. is only a relay station for sensory pathways

27. **Which of the following fibres terminate in the ventral posterior group of thalamic nuclei?**
    A. Medial lemniscus
    B. Spinal lemniscus
    C. Trigeminal lemniscus
    D. Solitariothalamic tract
    E. All the above

28. **Which of the following thalamic nuclei receives gustatory sensations?**
    A. Ventroposterior lateral nucleus
    B. Ventroposterior medial nucleus
    C. Ventral anterior nucleus
    D. Ventral intermediate nucleus
    E. Lateral dorsal nucleus

29. **The hypothalamus**
    A. forms the floor of interpeduncular fossa
    B. forms upper part of the lateral wall of the III ventricle

Ans. 24. A 25. B 26. D 27. E 28. B

C. is mainly made up of white matter

D. controls the activity of neurohypophysis through releasing hormones

E. is divided into medial and lateral zones by the internal capsule

30. The hypothalamus has all the following functions *except* that

A. it controls the activity of autonomic nervous system

B. it helps in regulating body temperature

C. it controls the activity of adenohypophysis through releasing hormones

D. it controls voluntary motor activity

E. it helps in regulating the circadian rythm

31. The epithalamus does *not* include the

A. pineal body

B. anterior commissure

C. habenular commissure

D. habenular nucleus

32. The auditory pathway does *not* include the

A. spiral ganglion

B. trapezoid body

C. medial lemniscus

D. inferior colliculus

E. medial geniculate body

33. The third ventricle

A. is the cavity of telencephalon

B. is bounded laterally by the medial surface of thalamus and hypothalamus separated by the hypothalamic sulcus

C. communicates anteroinferiorly with aqueduct cerebri

D. is closed superiorly (roofed) by the corpus callosum

E. communicates with the subarachnoid space through foramina of Luschka and Magendie

34. The caudate nucleus

A. forms part of paleostriatum

B. is named so because it lies caudal to the lentiform nucleus

C. sends its main efferents to cerebral cortex

D. is related to all parts of the lateral ventricle

E. has none of the above properties

Ans.   29. A   30. D   31. B   32. C   33. B   34. E

35. **The globus pallidus**
    A. is the darker medial part of the lentiform nuclcus
    B. forms the main efferent pathway for basal nuclei
    C. sends dopaminergic efferents to substantia nigra
    D. is mainly sensory in function
    E. has all the above features

36. **The medial surface of the cerebral hemisphere is supplied by the**
    A. anterior cerebral artery only
    B. anterior and middle cerebral arteries
    C. anterior and posterior cerebral arteries
    D. middle and posterior cerebral arteries
    E. anterior, middle and posterior cerebral arteries

37. **Which of the following sulci is present mainly on the superolateral surface of cerebral hemisphere?**
    A. Stem of lateral sulcus
    B. Parieto-occipital sulcus
    C. Calcarine sulcus
    D. Lunate sulcus
    E. Rhinal sulcus

38. **Motor speech area is located in the**
    A. superior frontal gyrus
    B. middle frontal gyrus
    C. inferior frontal gyrus
    D. medial frontal gyrus
    E. none of the above

39. **The auditory area**
    A. is located in the superior wall of posterior ramus of lateral sulcus
    B. is located in relation to superior temporal gyrus
    C. receives impulses from the contralateral ear only
    D. receives impulses from the ipsilateral ear only
    E. is supplied by the central branches of middle cerebral artery

40. **The visual area**
    A. is located in relation to the calcarine sulcus
    B. is mainly supplied by the middle cerebral artery

Ans.   35. B   36. C   37. D   38. C   39. B

C. has representation of macula in its most anterior part

D. receives fibres directly from the retina

E. receives optic radiation which arises from the medial geniculate body

41. The main efferents from the cerebellum arise from the
A. Purkinje cells
B. granule cells
C. Golgi cells
D. basket cells
E. cerebellar nuclei.

42. Most of the afferents to the cerebellum terminate in relation to the
A. Purkinje cells
B. granule cells
C. Golgi cells
D. basket cells
E. cerebellar nuclei

43. The archicerebellum
A. is represented only on the inferior aspect of cerebellum
B. develops late in the evolutionary history
C. is mainly concerned with maintenance of equillibrium
D. includes globose nucleus
E. is connected to the cerebrum through the cerebro-ponto-cerebellar pathway

44. The cerebellum is supplied by
A. internal carotid artery
B. vertebral artery
C. basilar artery
D. internal carotid and vertebral arteries
E. vertebral and basilar arteries

45. The cerebellar nuclei are arranged from lateral to medial side as
A. the dentate, the globose, the emboliform, the fastigial
B. the dentate, the emboliform, the globose and the fastigial
C. the fastigial, the globose, the emboliform and the dentate
D. the fastigial, the emboliform, the globose and the dentate

Ans.   40. A   41. E   42. A   43. C   44. E   45. B

46. **Functionally ventral horn cells are most closely related to**
    A. hypoglossal nucleus
    B. nucleus ambiguus
    C. dorsal nucleus of vagus
    D. facial nucleus

47. **Spinal nucleus of trigeminal nerve receives sensory fibres from which cranial nerves?**
    A. VI & VII
    B. VII & VIII
    C. VI & X
    D. VII & X

48. **The cell bodies of axons controlling voluntary activity of body on the opposite side are located in**
    A. ventral horn of spinal cord
    B. pre-central gyrus
    C. caudate nucleus
    D. dentate nucleus

49. **Which of the following cranial nerves contains axons of mesencephalic nucleus?**
    A. III
    B. V
    C. VII
    D. IX

50. **Which of the following nerves contains both general and special visceral efferent fibres**
    A. III
    B. V
    C. VII
    D. XII

51. **Medial geniculate body is associated with**
    A. vision
    B. hearing
    C. olfaction
    D. taste

52. **Cerebellum is associated with all the following *except***
    A. coordination of somatic motor activity

Ans.　46. A　47. D　48. B　49. B　50. C　51. B

    B. maintenance of tone of muscles

    C. integration of proprioception and reflex activity

    D. perception of tactile sensation

53. The main efferents of amygdaloid nucleus form

    A. fornix

    B. stria terminalis

    C. stria medullaris thalami

    D. tail of caudate nucleus

54. Which of the following structures does _not_ form part of pathway for recent memory?

    A. Hippocampus

    B. Fornix

    C. Septum pellucidum

    D. Mamillary body

55. Cerebrospinal fluid enters the cisterna magna from

    A. arachnoid granulations

    B. choroid plexus

    C. foramen of Magendie

    D. cistern of lateral sulcus

56. Injury to posterior column tracts of spinal cord will result into loss of

    A. pain sensation on same side

    B. temperature sensation on opposite side

    C. tactile discrimation on same side

    D. proprioceptive sensation on opposite side

57. Lesion of which tract results in positive Babinski sign?

    A. Rubrospinal

    B. Tectospinal

    C. Olivospinal

    D. Corticospinal

58. Flaccid paralysis with loss of tendon reflexes results from injury to

    A. corticospinal tract

    B. upper motor neuron

    C. ventral horn cells of spinal cord

    D. extrapyramidal pathways

Ans.   52. D   53. B   54. C   55. C   56. C   57. D   58. C

59. **Injury to lateral spinothalamic tract on one side results in loss of pain and temperature sensation**
    A. contralaterally one segment below the level of lesion
    B. contralaterally 2-3 segments below the level of lesion
    C. ipsilaterally one segment below the level of lesion
    D. ipsilaterally 2-3 segments below the level of lesion.

60. **Blockage at the level of aqueduct cerebri results in**
    A. enlargement of IV ventricle
    B. enlargement of lateral ventricles
    C. dilatation of subarachnoid cisterns
    D. dilatation of central canal of spinal cord

61. **A person is likely to burn his fingers while smoking in which of the following conditions?**
    A. Syringomyelia - degeneration around central canal of spinal cord
    B. Tabes dorsalis - involving dorsal roots
    C. Poliomyelites - involving ventral roots
    D. Hemisection of spinal cord.

62. **Lesions of archicerebellum is associated with**
    A. dysdiadocokinesia
    B. loss of equilibrium
    C. hemiplegia
    D. loss of reflexes

63. **Lesions of uncus are associated with**
    A. olfactory hallucinations
    B. visual hallucinations
    C. auditory hallucinations
    D. paraesthesias

64. **Symmetrical deficiency of pain and temperature sensation in both upper upper limbs is likely to be due to lesion of spinal cord involving**
    A. dorsal root
    B. spinothalamic tract
    C. anterior commissure
    D. posterior commissure

Ans.   59. A   60. B   61. A   62. B   63. A   64. C

65. **Bitemporal hemianopsia will result from injury to**
    A. middle part of optic chiasma
    B. optic tract
    C. optic radiation
    D. optic nerve

66. **Involvement of substantia nigra results in**
    A. nystagmus
    B. ataxia
    C. parkinsonism
    D. speech disturbances

67. **Hemiplegia with contralateral facial paralysis results from injury to**
    A. medulla oblongata
    B. pons-lower part
    C. pons-upper part
    D. mid brain

68. **Spastic paralysis in one half of body with contralateral inflanuclear paralysis of III cranial nerve results from involvement of**
    A. motor area of cortex
    B. internal capsule
    C. midbrain
    D. pons

69. **The pineal gland**
    A. is located in the groove between two inferior colliculi
    B. shows calcareous bodies called corpora amylacea
    C. it is attached to roof of III ventricle
    D. displacement of pineal shadow in a radiograph is an important sign of space occupying intracranial lesion.

70. **All the following statements are true for the 'Charcot' artery of cerebral haemorrhage** *except*
    A. is a central branch of anterior cerebral artery
    B. supplies internal capsule
    C. most commonly ruptured artery
    D. rupture results in hemiplegia on the opposite side

Ans.   65. A   66. C   67. B   68. C   69. D   70. A

71. **The premotor area shows all the following features** *except*
    A. located in posterior parts of superior, middle and inferior frontal gyri
    B. numbered as Brodmann's area 6
    C. main site for origin of pyramidal tracts
    D. lesion in this area results in impairment in performance of learned movements (apraxia)

72. **All the following statements pertaining to Broca's area are true** *except*
    A. located between horizontal and ascending ramus of lateral sulcus
    B. concerned with production of speech
    C. lesion results in paralysis of muscles involved in production of speech
    D. lesion of this area on right side in right handed individuals will not show much deficit.

73. **The internal capsule**
    A. has four parts
    B. genu lies between posterior limb and sublentiform part
    C. contains commissural fibres
    D. related laterally to lentiform nucleus.

74. **All the following statements pertain to internal capsule** *except*
    A. supplied by central branches of anterior and middle cerebral arteries
    B. small lesion causes widespread effects
    C. lesion in posterior limb results in contralateral hemiplegia and hemianaesthesia
    D. lesion of retrolentiform part results in auditory defects.

75. **Which of the following is a bundle of association fibres?**
    A. forceps major
    B. forceps minor
    C. cingulum
    D. fornix

76. **The characteristic features of Hydrocephalus include all the following** *except*
    A. proportionately large head

Ans.　71. C　72. C　73. D　74. D　75. C

   B. widening of sutures
   C. depressed anterior fontanellae
   D. bulging forehead (Frontal bossing)

77. **Blood-brain barrier consists of all the following** *except*
   A. endothelium of capillaries
   B. continuous basement membrane of capillaries
   C. epithelial cells of choroid plexus
   D. foot processes of astrocytes

78. **All the following statements pertain to subarachnoid haemorrhage** *except*
   A. commonly occurs due to rupture of aneurysm
   B. commonly occurs in interpeduncular cistern
   C. usually due to rupture of arteries of circle of Willis.
   D. lumbar puncture will not show blood stained C.S.F.

79. **Which of the following statements in relation to subdural haemorrhage is true**
   A. occurs under the endosteal layer of dura mater
   B. source of blood is from ruptured venous sinuses
   C. often extensive because of loose attachment of dura and arachnoid
   D. diagnosed by the presence of blood in C.S.F.

80. **Hemisection of spinal cord may result in all the following features below the level of injury** *except*
   A. complete loss of touch on opposite side
   B. loss of pain and temperature on opposite side
   C. spastic paralysis of muscles on same side
   D. loss of position sense on same side

Directions: For each of the incomplete statements or questions below, one or more completions or answers is correct. Select
   A. if only 1,2 and 3 are correct;
   B. if only 1 and 3 are correct;
   C. if only 2 and 4 are correct;
   D. if only 4 is correct;
   E. if all are correct.

Ans.   76. C   77. C   78. D   79. C   80. A

81. **The axon**
    1. begins at axon hillock which is rich in Nissl substance
    2. always allows impulses to travel in both directions
    3. is rich in ribosomes
    4. has smooth surface devoid of spines

82. **The muscle spindle**
    1. is a sensory end organ present in smooth muscle
    2. is innervated by gamma neurons
    3. has annulospiral nerve endings which terminate away from the equatorial region of intrafusal fibres
    4. provides information to the central nervous system about the extent and rate of stretching of the muscle

83. **In the region of the motor end plate**
    1. the axoplasm and the sarcoplasm become continuous with each other
    2. each axon terminal losses its myelin sheath
    3. sole plate is devoid of nuclei and mitochondria
    4. the transmitter is acetylcholine

84. **Which of the following statements is/are true for the spinal cord?**
    1. each spinal segment lies opposite the corresponding vertebra
    2. conus medullaris is continuous superiorly with medulla oblongata
    3. the anterior horn reaches close to the surface of the spinal cord
    4. the lateral horn is present only in the thoracic and upper lumbar segments

85. **The anterior corticospinal tract**
    1. is formed by axons arising from somatomotor as well as somatosensory cortex
    2. is a crossed tract
    3. terminates on the contralateral anterior horn cells of spinal cord
    4. extends throughout the spinal cord

86. **The rubrospinal tract**
    1. arises from the red nucleus

Ans.   81. D   82. C   83. C   84. D   85. B

   2. is a crossed tract
   3. descends in the lateral funiculus of spinal cord
   4. forms part of extrapyramidal system

87. The corticonuclear tract
   1. passes through the genu of internal capsule
   2. terminates in relation to all the efferent nuclei of various cranial nerves
   3. fibres mostly terminate in relation to nuclei of both sides
   4. injury leads to lower motor neuron type of paralysis

88. The lateral spinothalamic tract
   1. arises from the neurons in laminae VI, VII and VIII of the spinal cord
   2. fibres run obliquely for 3-4 segments before crossing
   3. carries pain and temperature sensations
   4. continues as lateral lemniscus in the pons

89. The anterior spinothalamic tract
   1. is made by up of first order neurons
   2. carries temperature sensation
   3. terminates in the anterior nucleus of thalamus
   4. is a crossed tract

90. Which of the following statements is/are true for medulla oblongata?
   1. Pyramids are paramedian elevations on its posterior aspect
   2. Olive lies ventromedial to the inferior cerebellar peduncle
   3. Its posterior surface forms whole of the floor of the IV ventricle
   4. Rootlets of vagus nerve are attached between olive and inferior cerebellar peduncle

91. At the level of the upper part of the olive, the medulla oblongata shows
   1. dorsal and ventral cochlear nuclei
   2. nucleus ambiguus
   3. nucleus of tractus solitarius
   4. hypoglossal nucleus

92. The olivary nucleus
   1. extends throughout the medulla oblongata

Ans.   86. E   87. A   88. B   89. D   90. C   91. E

2. sends its main efferents to contralateral cerebellar hemisphere
3. gives rise to mossy fibres of cerebellum
4. has a hilum directed dorsomedially

93. The medial lemniscus
1. is formed above the level of pyramidal decussation
2. consists of second order neurons carring proprioceptive impulses
3. forms a flat paramedian band just dorsal to the pyramid
4. ascends through the tectum of midbrain to terminate in ventro-posterior lateral nucleus of thalamus

94. Which of the following nuclei is/are connected with the IX cranial nerve?
1. Nucleus ambiguus
2. Inferior salivatory nucleus
3. Nucleus of tractus solitarius
4. Nucleus gracilis

95. The pons
1. lies dorsal to the cerebellum in the posterior cranial fossa
2. gives attachment to the trigeminal nerve on its ventral aspect
3. has a ventral tegmental part and a dorsal basilar part
4. is supplied by basilar artery

96. The lateral lemniscus
1. is formed in the medulla oblongata
2. is part of the hearing pathway
3. terminates in the superior colliculus
4. has both crossed and uncrossed fibres

97. The cochlear nuclei
1. represent second order neurons on auditory pathway
2. lie dorsal and ventral to the middle cerebellar peduncle
3. send efferents to form trapezoid body and lateral lemniscus
4. project to the auditory area of the opposite cerebral hemisphere only

98. The nuclei belonging to the special visceral efferent column in the pons are the
1. motor nucleus of trigeminal nerve

Ans. 92. C 93. A 94. A 95. C 96. C 97. B

    2. motor nucleus of abducent nerve
    3. motor nucleus of facial nerve
    4. superior salivatory nucleus

99. In relation to the midbrain
    1. it is a about 2 cm long
    2. tectum is the part between the cerebral aqueduct and the substantia nigra
    3. substantia nigra contains neurons rich in melanin pigment
    4. trochlear nerve is attached on the dorsal surface just cranial to the inferior colliculi

100. At the level of the superior colliculus, the features of midbrain include
    1. Edinger-Westphal nucleus
    2. red nucleus
    3. mesencephalic nucleus
    4. ventral tegmental decussation

101. The crura cerebri
    1. consist of fibres having origin in cerebral cortex
    2. are crossed laterally by the optic tracts
    3. are continuous inferiorly with the basilar part of pons
    4. are related to the oculomotor nerve medially

102. The superior colliculus
    1. receives fibres directly from retina
    2. is connected to the medial geniculate body through the superior brachium
    3. is a relay centre for visual reflexes
    4. is connected to the ipsilateral anterior horn cells through tectospinal tract

103. The features of thalamic nuclei include
    1. reticular nucleus lying in the internal medullary lamina
    2. intralaminar nuclei alter the level of alertness
    3. ventral anterior nucleus receives its main afferents from the hypothalamus
    4. anterior nucleus mainly projects to the cingulate gyrus

Ans. 98. B   99. B   100. A 101. E 102. B 103. C

104. **The hypothalamus**
    1. is divided into medial and lateral parts by the column of fornix and mamillothalamic tract
    2. controls the activity of adenohypophysis through hypo-thalamohypophyseal portal system
    3. is supplied by central branches of anterior and posterior cerebral arteries
    4. is related to the internal capsule laterally

105. **The neurohypophyseal hormones are produced by the**
    1. supraoptic nucleus
    2. preoptic nucleus
    3. paraventricular nucleus
    4. neurohypophysis itself

106. **The medial geniculate body**
    1. is purely a relay station on auditory pathway
    2. is connected to superior colliculus through superior brachium
    3. sends efferents to the ipsilateral auditory area
    4. has neurons arranged in six laminae

107. **The lateral geniculate body**
    1. lies at the upper end of the groove on the lateral aspect of midbrain
    2. receives impulses from the contralateral field of vision
    3. consists of neurons arranged in six laminae; the laminae 1,4 and 6 receiving fibres from the contralateral retina
    4. sends efferents to visual area through retrolentiform part of the internal capsule

108. **The third ventricle communicates**
    1. with the lateral ventricle through foramen of Monro
    2. with the aqueduct cerebri through foramen of Magendie
    3. with the fourth ventricle through aqueduct cerebri
    4. with the subarachnoid space through optic recess

109. **In relation to the lateral ventricle**
    1. the choroid plexus is present in all the parts
    2. the two lateral ventricles are separated by septum pellucidum
    3. the roof is formed by telachoroidea

Ans.   104. E 105. B 106. B 107. C 108. B

4. the medial wall of posterior horn shows two elevations; bulb of posterior horn and calcar avis

110. **In relation to the white matter of cerebral hemisphere**
 1. the commissural fibres connect corresponding parts of the two hemispheres
 2. the corpus callosum is made up of association fibres
 3. the anterior commissure mainly connects the olfactory areas of the two sides
 4. forceps minor connects occipital lobes of the two sides

111. **In relation to the motor area of cerebral cortex**
 1. it lies in the postcentral gyrus and extends on the medial surface into paracentral lobule
 2. any part of the body is represented by an area proportional to the size of the part
 3. the whole of motor area is supplied by the middle cerebral artery
 4. the body is represented upside down

112. **The corpus collosum**
 1. lies closer to the occipital pole as compared to the frontal pole
 2. is related throughout with the lateral ventricle
 3. is related superiorly to middle cerebral artery
 4. has some fibres which are not intersected by corona radiata

113. **The hippocampus**
 1. lies in the roof of the inferior horn of lateral ventricle
 2. has a posterior part called peshippocampus
 3. receives only olfactory impulses
 4. sends efferents to the mamillary body through the fornix

114. **The basal ganglia include**
 1. caudate nucleus
 2. lentiform nucleus
 3. claustrum
 4. red nucleus

115. **The reticular formation**
 1. consists of a diffuse network of fibres only
 2. consists of multisynaptic pathway

Ans. 109. C 110. B 111. D 112. C 113. D 114. A

    3. is confined to hind brain

    4. influences the level of consciousness and alertness

116. The general visceral efferent nuclei of the brainstem does *not* include

    1. Edinger-Westphal nucleus

    2. motor nucleus of fifth nerve

    3. lacrimatory nucleus

    4. nucleus ambiguus

117. The nucleus of tractus solitarius

    1. lies in the floor of IV ventricle

    2. is concerned with taste sensations

    3. receives fibres from V, VII and IX cranial nerves

    4. gives efferents which form solitariothalamic tract

118. The functional components of vagus nerve include

    1. general visceral efferent fibres arising from the dorsal nucleus

    2. general somatic afferent fibres terminating in the spinal nucleus of trigeminal nerve

    3. special visceral afferent fibres terminating in the nucleus of solitary tract

    4. somatic efferent fibres arising from the nucleus ambiguus

119. In relation to the visual pathway

    1. fibres arising from one retina go to the lateral geniculate body of that side only

    2. fibres carrying visual impulses from the temporal field of vision cross in the optic chiasma

    3. optic radiation passes through the sublentiform part of internal capsule

    4. upper half of field of vision is represented in the lower part of visual area of cortex

120. In relation to the nuclei of trigeminal nerve

    1. they extend from the midbrain to the upper part of spinal cord

    2. the main sensory nucleus in concerned with proprioceptive impulses

    3. the mesencephalic nucleus has unipolar neurons

    4. the spinal nucleus gives efferents to form spinal tract of trigeminal nerve

Ans. 115. C 116. B 117. C 118. A 119. C 120. A

Directions: Each question consists of an assertion and a reason. Answers should be choosen as follows:

    A. if the assertion and reason are true statements and the reason is a correct explanation of the assertion;

    B. if the assertion and reason are true statements but the reason is not a correct explanation of the assertion;

    C. if the assertion is true but the reason is a false statement;

    D. if the assertion is false but the reason is a true statement;

    E. if both assertion and reason are false statements.

121. **The posterolateral herniation of intervertebral disc at cervicothoracic junction will affect size of the pupil**
Because
the first thoracic nerve will be compressed

122. **The thoracic region of the spinal cord is most susceptible to ischaemia**
Because
there is an additional lateral horn in this region

123. **In case of raised intracranial tension, the cerebrospinal fluid should be rapidly removed**
Because
removal of cerebrospinal fluid will temporarily relieve pressure on the brain.

124. **In tabes dorsalis, which involves dorsal roots of spinal nerves, there is no change in muscle tone**
Because
the dorsal roots are purely sensory in function

125. **In syringomyelia the patient usually has bilateral segmental loss of pain and thermal sensibility**
Because
the crossing fibres of anterior spinothalmic tract are destroyed

126. **Lumbar puncture should be done between L1 and L2 vertebrae**
Because
the spinal cord usually ends at this level

Ans.   121. E 122. E 123. D 124. D 125. C 126. D

127. **In medial medullary syndrome there occurs hemiparesis, loss of touch and proprioceptive sensations and paralysis of muscles of tongue on the opposite side of body**
Because
there is involvement of pyramids, medial lemniscus and hypoglossal nerve on that side

128. **Thrombosis of anterior cerebral artery on the medial surface of cerebral hemisphere will result in contralateral hemiplegia**
Because
motor area extends on to the medial surface of the cerebral hemisphere

129. **A small haemorrhage in the region of internal capsule produces widespread paralysis of the opposite half of the body**
Because
all motor fibres to the opposite half of the body lie in a small area occupying the genu and posterior limb of internal capsule

130. **Lesions of one cerebellar hemisphere give rise to signs and symptoms that are limited to the opposite half of the body**
Because
one cerebellar hemisphere receives fibres from the opposite cerebral hemisphere

131. **Injury to the optic chiasma results in the loss of vision in both the nasal halves of the fields of vision**
Because
in the optic chiasma fibres arising from the nasal halves of both retinae cross.

132. **In Argyll-Robertson pupil, the light reflex persists while pupillary reaction to accommodation reflex is gone**
Because
the two pathways separate beyond the lateral geniculate body

133. **Blockage of aqueduct leads to hydrocephalus**
Because
exit of cerebrospinal fluid from the lateral and third ventricles is blocked

Ans.   127. D 128. D 129. A 130. D 131. D 132. D 133. A

134. **If hemiplegia is associated with ptosis and lateral squint the injury is most likely to be at the level of pons**
Because
abducent nerve which supplies the lateral rectus muscle has its origin in the pons

135. **A symmetrical loss of sensation of pain and temperature in both the forefingers suggests a lesion in the anterior white commissure of spinal cord**
Because
the fibres in the lateral spinothalamic tracts cross over in the anterior white commissure

Ans.   134. D 135. A